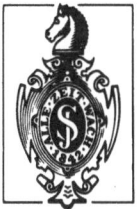

Frank Horan · Peter Beighton

Orthopaedic Problems in Inherited Skeletal Disorders

Foreword by W. J. W. Sharrard

With 98 Figures

Springer-Verlag
Berlin Heidelberg New York 1982

Frank Horan, MSc, FRCS
Consultant Orthopaedic Surgeon
Cuckfield Hospital, Cuckfield
Sussex, England

Peter Beighton, MD, PhD, FRCP, DCH
Professor of Human Genetics
Medical School and Groote Schuur Hospital
University of Cape Town
Cape, South Africa

ISBN-13: 978-1-4471-1328-7   e-ISBN-13: 978-1-4471-1326-3
DOI: 10.1007/978-1-4471-1326-3

Filmset by Polyglot Pte Ltd, Singapore
Printed by Butler & Tanner Ltd, Frome and London

2128/3916-543210

In memory of our fathers, for the example
which they set to us when we were young

Foreword

Inherited skeletal disorders have a fascination for many medical and surgical disciplines. For the geneticist there is interest in the study of families and their inheritance of lesions. The paediatrician is concerned because most of the disorders present in childhood as a problem in clinical differential diagnosis. The radiologist is interested because of the manifest, multiple and curious bone changes that provide a challenge in diagnosis and classification. The orthopaedic surgeon is involved because they present a challenge in the management of the many and various lesions of the limbs and trunk.

Most of the text books are slanted towards one or other aspect of the subject, depending upon the specialist interests of their author. Though informative to colleagues in their own discipline, the information which they contain is liable to be overwhelming in its complexity or unhelpful in its content for the orthopaedic surgeon or trainee.

Frank Horan and Peter Beighton have aimed their admirable and concise monograph to help the orthopaedic surgeon—the one individual who is likely to be able to ameliorate the musculo-skeletal problems from which so many of the children and adults with these diseases suffer. In recent years, much more orthopaedic help has become available for dysplastics. Improvements in technique and understanding have provided cervical spine fusions for atlanto-axial defects, spine corrections and fusions for scoliosis and kypho-scoliosis, multiple osteotomies and expandable rods for the treatment of osteogenesis imperfecta, corrective bony and soft tissue procedures for limb defects, limb lengthening for short limbs and joint replacements for adults with secondary arthritis. I feel sure that this book will be immensely helpful to the individual orthopaedic surgeon by indicating to him what he can offer to the dysplastic. The orthopaedic trainee will have up-to-date and readable information to supplement the knowledge that he needs to acquire during his training. It is not too much to hope that here and there, there may be orthopaedic surgeons who will be inspired to join with their colleagues in other disciplines to try to find further solutions to the problems and difficulties which so many dysplastics have to face.

Sheffield, February 1982

W.J.W. Sharrard
MD, ChM, FRCS

Preface

The striking appearance of some inherited abnormalities of the skeleton has been a source of fascination since the Middle Ages, and the dramatic descriptions of such disorders which appeared in the early medical literature were usually couched in terms of hyperbole and bewilderment. Before the publication in 1951 of Sir Thomas Fairbank's classic 'Atlas of General Affections of the Skeleton' there was no comprehensive monograph to which the surgeon could turn for enlightenment and guidance. More recently a number of books have appeared in which current knowledge is summarised and classified, but although they contain detailed descriptive, radiographic and genetic information, views on the management of the syndromes described are usually dealt with only briefly.

We have written this book for the practising orthopaedic surgeon. It is based on our experience with more than 1000 patients whose details are recorded in the Bone Dysplasia Registry of the Department of Human Genetics, University of Cape Town, together with numerous others studied in the United Kingdom and North America during the past 15 years.

A general outline of the basic principles of clinical genetics and the problems of classification of these disorders is given in the early chapters. The principal clinical and radiological features of the more common conditions are then described and illustrated. We have made a special effort to include an account of the medical and surgical treatment which is now available. The genetic aspects of the syndromes are discussed only briefly since we consider that the problems of counselling are best dealt with by clinical geneticists who have special experience of this difficult task.

We have restricted references in the text to contemporary views on the syndromes and to their clinical management. The standard monographs which provide fuller syndrome description and discuss radiology and genetics in more detail are listed separately.

This book is not intended to be comprehensive, but includes accounts of the more common and clinically important members of this rare group of disorders.

January 1982   Frank Horan
                                                               Peter Beighton

Acknowledgements

We have received assistance in many shapes and forms and we wish to express our thanks to those who have been involved in our endeavours:

To Sonia Brookes, Gillian Shapley and Barbara Breytenbach of Cape Town and Lorna Blurton of Cuckfield for patiently typing the manuscript;

To R. A. de Méneaud and C. Russ for preparing many of the illustrations;

To our colleagues Bryan Cremin, George Dall and Brookes Heywood of Cape Town, Herman Hamersma of Pretoria and André Bathfield and Louis Solomon of Johannesburg for access to clinical and radiographic material;

To Drs. R. O. Murray, H. A. Sissons and D. J. S. Stoker for encouraging our studies of the Fairbank Collection in the Radiology Museum of the Institute of Orthopaedics, London;

To genetic nursing sisters and cripple care nurses, past and present – Lecia Durr, Elizabeth Napier, Rosemary Duggan, Lorraine Groeneveldt, Gail Barnard, Meriel Macrae and Sue Dunstan of Cape Town and Pam Otto, Ann Williams and Judith Mathee of Johannesburg;

To the South African Medical Research Council and the University of Cape Town Staff Research Fund for financial support for our investigations of the skeletal dysplasias;

To Michael Jackson of Springer-Verlag for his support and hospitality and for the benign tolerance with which he gently guided us to our deadline.

Contents

1. Genetic Principles

Genetic principles and their application to orthopaedics are briefly reviewed in this chapter and relevant technical terms are explained. This summary is necessarily very superficial, and for a more detailed account of basic genetics reference should be made to the monograph 'Elements of Medical Genetics' (Emery 1979).

1.1 Basic Genetics

The cell nucleus consists almost entirely of deoxyribose nucleic acid (DNA), which aggregates into chromosomes at cell division. Each human somatic cell contains 46 chromosomes, 23 of which have been derived from each parent. One pair of chromosomes which are concerned with the determination of biological sex, are known as the 'sex chromosomes', while the remaining 44 chromosomes are termed 'autosomes'.

The chromosomes have short and long arms (designated 'p' and 'q' respectively) and the point of union of these components is the centromere. The 23 pairs are conveniently numbered on the basis of their morphological configuration. Precise identification of an individual chromosome in the laboratory has been facilitated by recent developments in staining techniques, which allow the demonstration of patterns of transverse banding.

The DNA molecule has a double helical shape and may be regarded as resembling a step ladder which has been twisted upon itself. A few steps of this molecular ladder constitute a gene, of which there are many thousands on each chromosome. Genes are highly specific in both their action and their topographical location on any particular chromosome. The genetic constitution of any individual is known as the 'genotype', while the clinical manifestations of gene action are termed the 'phenotype'.

1.2 Chromosomal Disorders

Chromosomes are visible by light microscopy in suitably prepared specimens of cultured white cells or other tissues, and in a few disorders numerical or structural chromosomal aberrations can be detected in this way. However, in most heritable conditions the defect lies in an abnormality of the genes and cytogenetic studies will prove unrewarding. Although a few syndromes caused by chromosomal abnormalities have significant orthopaedic complications these afflictions are rare and usually fatal in infancy.

1.3 Gene Disorders

As one member of each of the 23 pairs of chromosomes has been derived from each parent, the genes themselves may be considered to be paired. An individual with a pair of similar genes is regarded as being 'homozygous' for that particular trait and is termed a 'homozygote', while a person with a pair of dissimilar genes is termed a 'heterozygote'.

Conditions which are the consequence of faulty genes are conventionally classified in terms of the mode of inheritance within a kindred. The following broad groups are recognised:

1.3.1 Autosomal Dominant

An autosomal dominant disorder is a result of a single faulty gene and males and females are affected in equal proportions. The condition is transmitted from generation to generation and there is a 50% risk that any offspring of an affected individual will receive the gene (Fig. 1.1).

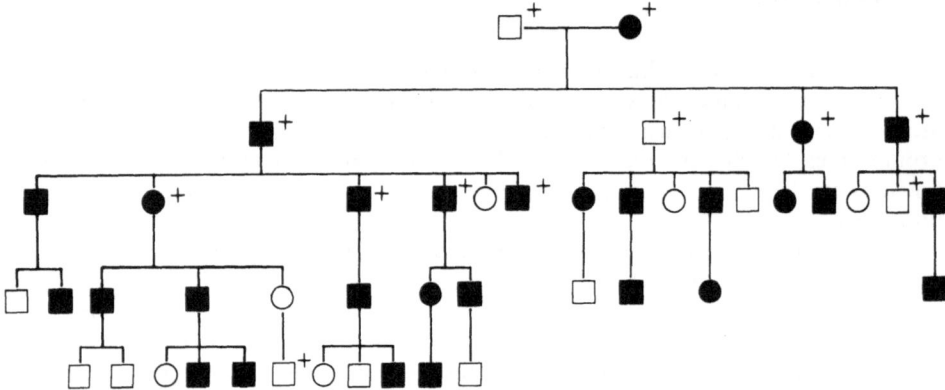

Fig. 1.1. Autosomal dominant inheritance in familial generalised joint hypermobility. ■, male, affected; □, male, unaffected; ●, female, affected; ○, female, unaffected; +, deceased.

In kindreds with an autosomal dominant trait an affected person may have normal parents. This is usually the consequence of a new mutation of the abnormal gene in the gonad of one or other parent. Mutation has been shown to be associated with advanced paternal age in a number of dominant conditions such as achondroplasia and the Marfan syndrome, and it is likely that a similar effect will be demonstrated in other less common disorders which are of orthopaedic significance once sufficient clinical and pedigree data has been accumulated.

1.3.2 Autosomal Recessive

Autosomal recessive disease is the result of homozygosity for a pair of faulty genes and several hundred genetic disorders are inherited by this mechanism. In a kindred with an autosomal recessive condition the parents will be clinically normal although they will both be heterozygous for the gene in question. Theoretically there is a one in four chance that any child produced by these parents will inherit both faulty genes and be homozygous for, and therefore have, the condition. There is also a one in four chance that the child will not inherit any faulty genes and a two in four chance that he will have one normal and one faulty gene, in which case he would be heterozygous for the condition, like his parents, and would be clinically normal but be genetically a carrier. Many disorders which are of orthopaedic importance show this pattern of inheritance, and a pedigree of such a kindred with the Schwartz syndrome (blepharophimosis, myotonia, skeletal deformity and dwarfism) is shown in Fig. 1.2.

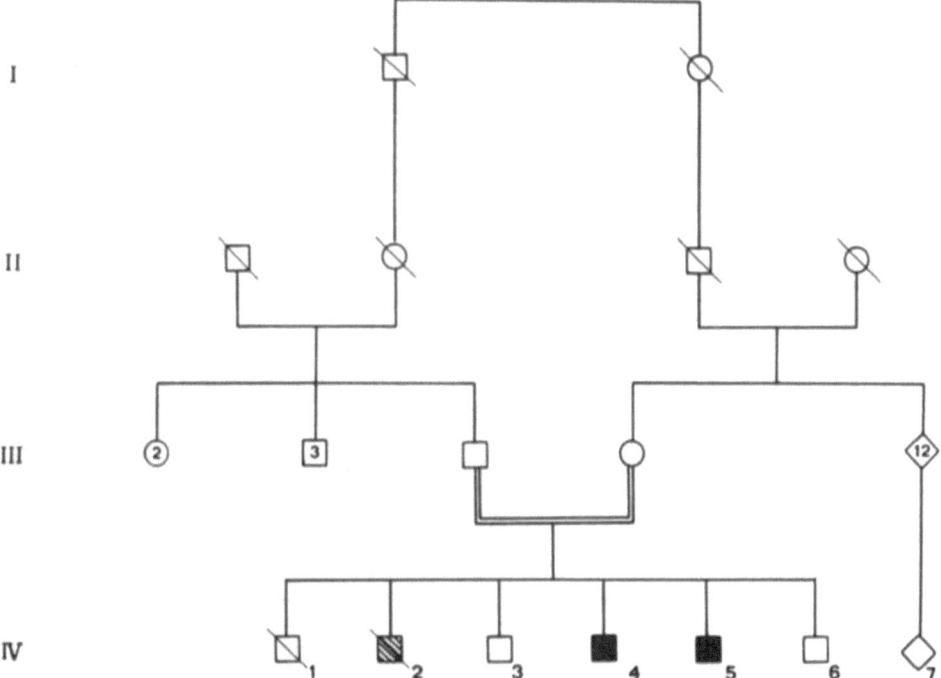

Fig. 1.2. Autosomal recessive inheritance in the Schwartz syndrome. ■, male, affected; □, male, unaffected; ●, female, affected; ○, female, unaffected; ▨, male, thought to be affected, not examined; ◇, sex unknown, not examined; ＼, deceased.

The likelihood of both parents being heterozygous for the same faulty gene is greatly increased if they share a similar genetic constitution by virtue of being related to each other, and therefore consanguineous marriages, such as those between cousins, have an increased chance of producing offspring with autosomal recessive disease.

1.3.3 X-Linked Inheritance

In X-linked conditions the responsible gene is carried on the X chromosome and the condition is manifest only in the male. An affected male cannot pass the trait on to his sons since he gives them his unaffected Y chromosome, but he will transmit his X chromosome bearing the abnormal gene to all his daughters, who will then be asymptomatic carriers of the disorder.

Carrier females can transmit an X chromosome carrying either a faulty or a normal gene to both daughters and sons; the sons who receive the gene develop the disease, while the daughters remain asymptomatic carriers. Examples of X-linked recessive bone dysplasias are the Hunter syndrome (mucopolysaccharidosis type II) and spondyloepiphyseal dysplasia tarda (Fig. 1.3).

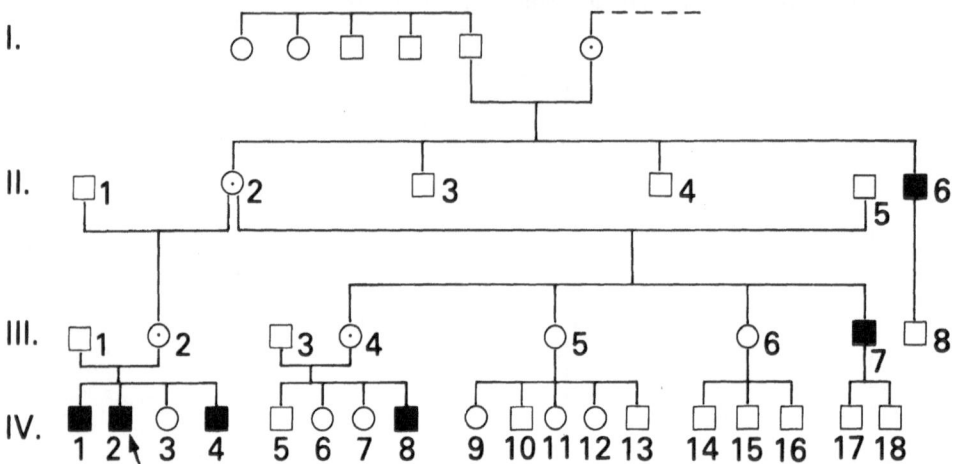

Fig. 1.3. Pedigree of a patient with X-linked recessive form of the Ehlers-Danlos syndrome.

X-linked dominant conditions are very few in number and vitamin D-resistant rickets is the only skeletal syndrome in this category which is likely to be encountered. In this type of inheritance the disorder is manifest in both male and female heterozygotes. The male transmits the trait to all his daughters but none of his sons, while the female is at risk of passing the disease to half of her children irrespective of their sex.

1.3.4 Polygenic Inheritance

Polygenic inheritance is a complex process and the clinical stigmata in conditions of this type are the result of the action of a cluster of faulty genes. An environmental determinant may also be involved and in these circumstances the disorder is regarded as being 'multifactorial' in aetiology. In a kindred with a polygenic or multifactorial condition the risks of recurrence are much higher than in the population as a whole. For instance, in the neural tube defects or in congenital talipes equinovarus there is approximately a 5% (1 in 20) risk of recurrence in any subsequent sibling after an affected child has been born. However, there is no characteristic pattern of distribution within the family.

Reference

Emery AEH (1979) Elements of medical genetics, 5th edn., Churchill Livingstone, Edinburgh

2. The Investigation and General Management of Bone Dysplasias

The correct diagnosis of a bone dysplasia may require the interpretation of clinical, family, radiographic, and biochemical data. Clinical examination will usually establish the presence of abnormality, but precise delineation of the condition may require further extensive investigation.

2.1 Assessment of the Patient

2.1.1 Clinical Examination

Many bone dysplasias may be recognised clinically because of their unique characteristics. During routine examination the facies and body build are carefully inspected and the height, span, and upper and lower body segments are measured. In normal circumstances the segments from crown to pubis and from pubis to heel are of equal length. Bone dysplasias which are characterised by a general retardation in growth affect height more than span, while disparity between long bone and vertebral growth or alignment will be revealed by segment measurement.

Limb length discrepancy and the relative length of limb segments are then assessed and the hands and feet are inspected for abnormality of structure. The joints are examined for congruity and mobility.

In some skeletal dysplasia syndromes involvement of non-osseous structures may provide a diagnostic clue. A general examination of all systems is undertaken, with emphasis on the skin, hair, nails, and eyes. Finally, visual and auditory acuity are determined and intelligence and the degree of mental development are assessed.

2.1.2 Genealogical Studies

A careful study of the kindred must be undertaken and a family tree, or pedigree, drawn up in order to evaluate the genetic aspects of the disorder. Ideally, information concerning all known relatives should be obtained and as many family members as possible examined. The clinical manifestations of a syndrome may vary between individuals and generations within the same family.

2.1.3 Radiological Assessment

All bone disorders show radiological abnormalities. Some conditions may be strictly localised but many involve the whole skeleton, and it is therefore usual to undertake a skeletal survey of affected persons. Radiographic examination of relatives may be necessary, but the extent of these investigations will vary according to the syndrome involved. Minor radiological changes may be the only detectable abnormality in relatives in whom the gene is incompletely expressed, or in some heterozygous carriers of recessive disorders.

2.1.4 Biochemical Investigation

Some skeletal abnormalities are the consequence of genetically determined enzymatic deficiencies. These biochemical disorders are usually inherited as autosomal recessive traits and the majority are characterised by the accumulation of metabolic products which have been incompletely broken down. These abnormal metabolites may be excreted in the urine, where their detection can provide the key to the diagnosis of the syndrome. The mucopolysaccharidoses are a good example, as defective enzymatic activity in these disorders leads to the storage and urinary excretion of incompletely degraded glycosaminoglycans. The diagnosis of the individual mucopolysaccharidosis is usually suspected on recognition of the characteristic clinical and radiographic features and subsequently confirmed by the identification of the abnormal substances in the urine. The specific enzyme deficiency in the majority of mucopolysaccharidoses may be accurately determined by studies of cultured fibroblasts.

2.2 Other Investigations

2.2.1 Radio-isotope Scanning of Bone

An increase in uptake of radio-isotopes such as technetium^{99m} can be demonstrated in the presence of increased bone blood flow or metabolic turnover. This is rarely found in uncomplicated bone dysplasias, although an increase in uptake of radio-isotopes has been observed in melorheostosis. Nevertheless, bone scans may be useful in differentiating skeletal dysplasias from infection or neoplasia. Dysplasias which have a potential for the development of malignancy may be monitored by isotope scans. Epstein and Levin (1978) have described the successful detection of neoplastic change in hereditary multiple exostoses by this technique.

2.2.2 Computerised Tomography

Computerised tomography has been used to assess the progress of bone dysplasias, particularly those involving the spine. This procedure has been of considerable value in depicting the structure of the spinal canal in patients with achondroplasia who have developed symptoms which are suggestive of spinal stenosis (Fig. 2.1).

2.2.3 Histological Studies

Histological and electron microscopic examination of biopsy specimens of bone and cartilage from persons with skeletal dysplasias are of diagnostic value in a few rare conditions, but such investigations do not have a wide application at present.

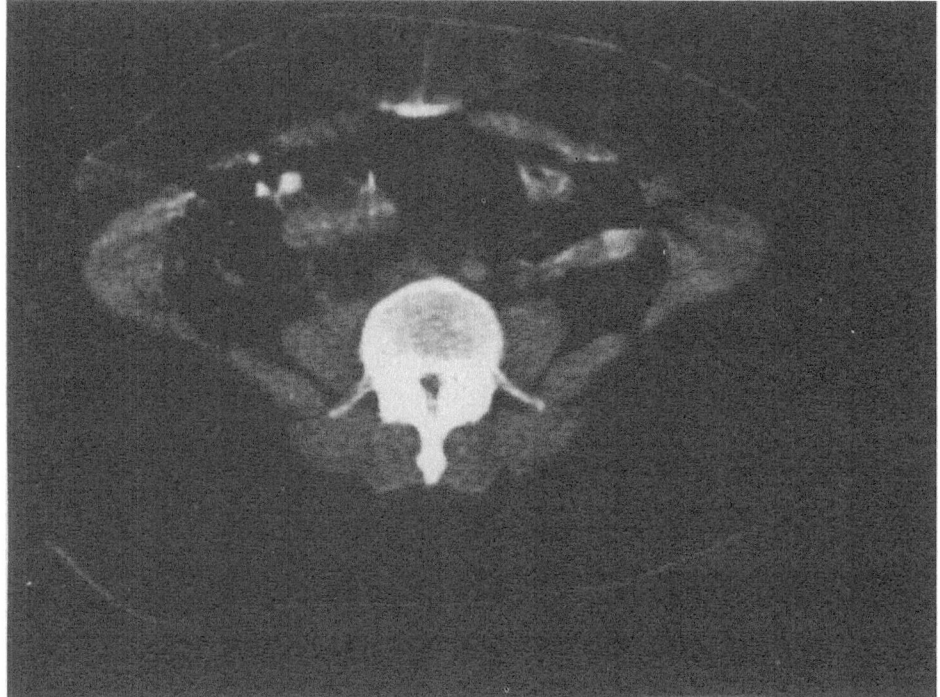

Fig. 2.1. CT scan of fourth lumbar vertebra in achondroplasia.

2.2.4 Histochemical Studies

Histochemical examination of cultured fibroblasts has been used for diagnostic and research purposes. Abnormalities of collagen ultrastructure have been recognised in a few connective tissue disorders, such as certain forms of the Ehlers-Danlos syndrome and osteogenesis imperfecta.

2.3 Antenatal Diagnosis

Antenatal diagnosis is a rapidly growing facet of clinical genetics which is becoming increasingly important in the management of skeletal dysplasias.

2.3.1 Amniocentesis

In this technique a specimen of amniotic fluid is aspirated from the gravid uterus about 16 weeks after conception. Cytogenetic abnormalities in the foetus may be detected in cultured amniotic cells, while a number of biochemical abnormalities can be recognised by studies of the metabolic activity of these cells. Other conditions, notably meningocoele and anencephaly, produce a raised level of alpha-fetoprotein in the amniotic fluid; maternal serum alpha-fetoprotein concentrations are also elevated, and maternal serum screening is now a routine procedure in many centres as an initial step in the detection of foetal neural tube defects.

2.3.2 Foetoscopy

Foetoscopy enables examination of the foetus through an optical system which is attached to a needle inserted into the gravid uterus. In a few disorders the pregnancy may be monitored by means of foetal blood sampling, which is carried out by placental needling or by puncture of a placental blood vessel under direct vision at foetoscopy. At present these techniques play only a small part in antenatal diagnosis, but it may be anticipated that their role will increase in the future.

2.3.3 Antenatal Radiography

Although radiation to the foetus must be avoided if possible, radiography is valuable in the diagnosis and assessment of skeletal dysplasia in the last trimester of pregnancy (Cremin and Beighton 1978).

2.3.4 Ultrasonography

Abnormalities such as anencephaly, hydrocephaly and spinal dysraphism can be detected in early pregnancy by ultrasonography (Kossof et al. 1974). The field is developing very rapidly and sophisticated techniques such as grey-scale ultrasonography allow more accurate definition of the foetus.

2.3.5 General Considerations

The majority of monitored pregnancies will be shown to be normal and antenatal diagnosis will then provide reassurance for parents with a foetus which is potentially 'at risk'. However, before investigation, the medical geneticist and the parents will have had to agree to termination of the pregnancy if the unborn child proves to be abnormal.

2.4 The General Management of Bone Dysplasias

The management of individual disorders will be reviewed in later chapters, but it is pertinent to discuss the topic in general terms.

Bone dysplasias are rare and consequently there are few centres with staff who are experienced in their management. The variety of problems posed may require a team approach with involvement of specialists such as a medical geneticist, a paediatrician, an orthopaedic surgeon, a neurosurgeon, an ear, nose and throat surgeon, an orthotist, a prosthetist, and social workers.

Accuracy of diagnosis is essential before an informed prognosis and correct genetic counselling can be given and a proper programme of management arranged. It may be necessary to observe the patient for some time, particularly in infancy or early childhood, before the full features of the syndrome have become manifest. There is usually no need to reach a hasty decision and caution is always warranted. Careful thought, appraisal of the relevant literature, and consultation with interested colleagues will assist in the diagnosis of a difficult case.

2.4.1 Psycho-social Problems

Parents of affected children need skilled and sympathetic handling. Their world may have been shattered by an event which is quite outside their experience and of which they have little understanding. They may reject the diagnosis and its implications. Certainly they will need to be made gradually aware of the probable outcome for their child and of its likely handicaps. In view of the possibility of future pregnancy the most informed and experienced genetic counselling must be made available to assuage parental worry.

In general, when a bone dysplasia is first diagnosed in an adult the prognosis is much brighter and the psycho-social problems are correspondingly less. However, assistance may be needed in social and work adjustment, and the establishment of an understanding relationship between patient and surgeon is vital.

2.4.2 General Considerations

Few bone dysplasias can be cured, so the main aim of management is to make the best use of available function and to prevent or minimise further disability. A realistic assessment must be made of the physical and mental potential of the patient. It is self-evident that extensive surgery or attempts to prolong the life of an infant or young child in whom early death can be accurately forecast are unwarranted.

Braces, splints and collars have their place in conservative management, but their bulk and weight may be too much for a child whose physical and mechanical function are already seriously impaired. Care must be taken to ensure that the patient is not made less mobile by misguided attempts to hold him straight or support his limbs. Appliances require skilled manufacture and careful fitting and need continual surveillance, since even dwarfed children may grow and change their shape at a surprising rate.

Surgical operations are being used increasingly to prevent deformity, to improve both the appearance and function of an established malformation, and to deal with potentially dangerous problems which may result from abnormal growth. The results of operation are, on the whole, satisfactory in skilled hands. Even so, relapse and recurrence of a deformity often occur and the surgeon and patient must be prepared for revision procedures, particularly in children, until they have exhausted their potential for growth. The patient, the relatives and the surgeon must each understand the aim of the operation before it is undertaken, so that disappointment and resentment do not occur if a 'perfect' result is not achieved.

2.4.3 Dwarfism

When considering the operative management of dwarfism it is wise to recall quotations from two notable authorities on the subject. Bailey (1973) in the preface to his book 'Disproportionate Short Stature' remarked that many such patients who were seen by him said, 'I was doing alright until they operated on me'. Kopits (1976) opened his review of the orthopaedic complications of dwarfism with the sentence, 'The most significant problem with dwarfs is not so much their shortness of stature as the medical problems complicating their basic condition.'

Dwarfs are short because of the inherent defects in their mechanism for skeletal growth. Their short stature may be made worse by additional skeletal deformity such as scoliosis or lower limb abnormality and skilled management may help prevent or lessen these secondary problems. Early operative correction and fusion for scoliosis is being undertaken more frequently. A number of surgeons are now performing leg-lengthening procedures in achondroplasts and other short-limbed dwarfs and, although such operations may present considerable hazards, their advocates claim that the results are worth the risks involved.

Signs of cord compression may result from spinal stenosis, as in the lumbar spine in achondroplasts, a fixed kyphosis, or from atlanto-axial instability, which may occur in dysplasias in which odontoid hypoplasia is a feature, in particular the Morquio syndrome, spondyloepiphyseal dysplasia (S.E.D.) congenita, and pseudo-achondroplasia. Perovic et al. (1973) claimed that 75% of non-achondroplastic dwarfs had atlanto-axial instability and that more than 50% of these patients had cervical myelopathy, but these figures may well be high. In such cases great care must be taken when anaesthetics are administered because of the danger of damage to the cervical cord.

2.4.4 The Lower Limbs

The management of disorders of weight-bearing joints and the lower limbs should be based on the accepted orthopaedic principle of the maintenance of mechanical alignment when standing and walking, since failure to achieve this may result in abnormal ligament stress and early degenerative change in the knee, subluxation of the hip, pelvic tilt, and scoliosis. Dysplasia of the developing hip may require upper femoral or pelvic osteotomy. Arthrography may be necessary for the assessment of the state of the hip joint in the growing child.

The fully developed hip joint may be discongruous and pain and disability will develop early if there are premature degenerative changes affecting the articular surface. Replacement arthroplasty of these hips has been very successful but the operation may present considerable technical difficulty. The size and configuration of the acetabulum and upper end of the femur may require prostheses of small size and varied shape, and careful radiographic evaluation of the available bone stock must be made when the operation is being planned. Skilled anaesthesia is mandatory as intubation may be difficult, and tracheostomy may be necessary.

Malalignment of the knees may warrant corrective osteotomy and replacement arthroplasty has been successful in patients with disabling arthritic changes.

In considering the management of foot problems the only reasonable criterion is that of function. Operation should not be undertaken until the full range of supports, insoles, and special footwear has been exhausted in attempts to preserve painless weight-bearing. It should be born in mind that foot deformities in children tend to relapse after operation, although the outlook is less gloomy in adults.

The care of patients with bone dysplasias is a lifetime commitment for both the surgeon and the patient. A successful outcome depends upon a careful appraisal of the condition with an attitude of judicious optimism and mutual respect in both parties.

2.4.5 Genetic Counselling

Genetic counselling involves the discussion of the clinical pattern and the risk of recurrence with an individual with an inherited disease or the parents of an affected child. Success is dependent upon diagnostic precision which, in turn, may require the full range of investigations outlined earlier in this chapter.

It is a fundamental tenet of genetic practice that the patient must make the final decision concerning any action, although it is the duty of the genetic counsellor to provide all the relevant information. The actual magnitude of risk of recurrence is often overshadowed by the potential clinical consequences of the disorder. Thus the 'burden of the disease' is very great in a condition such as diastrophic dysplasia, where there is gross dwarfism and skeletal distortion, in comparison with talipes equinovarus which may be rectified surgically.

Genetic counselling is not a job for the inexperienced, and patients or parents who require such advice must be referred to a specialist genetic clinic.

References

Bailey JA II (1973) Disproportionate short stature. Saunders, Philadelphia London Toronto

Cremin BJ, Beighton P (1978) Bone dysplasias of infancy. Springer, Berlin Heidelberg New York

Epstein DA, Levin EJ (1978) Bone scintigraphy in hereditary multiple exostoses. Am J Roentgenol 130:331

Kopits SE (1976) Orthopaedic complications of dwarfism. Clin Orthop 114:153

Kossoff G, Garrett WJ, Rodovanovich G (1974) Grey scale echography in obstetrics and gynaecology. Aust Radiol 18:63

Perovic MN, Kopits SE, Thompson RC (1973) Radiological evaluation of the spinal canal in congenital atlanto-axial dislocation. Radiology 109:713

3. Nomenclature and Terminology

3.1 Introduction

The majority of the inherited skeletal dysplasias are rare, and until recently they have been grouped into general categories rather than delineated into specific disorders. The realisation that the recognition and accurate definition of individual abnormalities facilitates satisfactory management and prognostication, has led to increased efforts towards the separation and precise identification of individual syndromes.

The disorders in which disproportionate dwarfism occurs provide an excellent example of the development of concepts concerning syndromic identity. In the past short-limbed dwarfs tended to be grouped together as achondroplasts or 'achondroplasia variants' without any further attempt at diagnostic accuracy. The alternative term 'osteochondrodysplasia' was sometimes employed and although this allusion to the underlying defect represented a step towards a scientific basis for identification, it was still non-specific. During the past two decades interest has been focused on these disorders and numerous disease entities have now been delineated from this previously amorphous group.

As clinical, radiographic, biochemical and genetic information accumulates it is becoming apparent that conditions which were regarded as specific syndromes are, in fact, separate disorders which may only have a superficial resemblance to each other. Considerable residual heterogeneity remains and the development and application of new techniques of investigation will permit further sub-categorisation.

3.2 Historical Perspectives

Sir Thomas Fairbank of the Royal National Orthopaedic Hospital, London, laid the foundation for many present-day concepts concerning the inherited bone dysplasias. During an illustrious medical career which spanned 50 years and encompassed the Anglo-Boer War, the Great War and World War II, Sir Thomas' interest in these conditions resulted in the accumulation of a considerable amount of clinical and radiographic material, which is now stored in the museum of the Department of Radiology at the Institute of Orthopaedics. Sir Thomas' classic 'Atlas of General Affections of the Skeleton' was based upon these data. The development of his ideas concerning separate disease entities is readily evident in the successive editions of his book, and in the meticulous annotations which he made on the case notes and radiographs in the collection. It is an enriching experience to read these comments and to trace the emergence of specific syndromes.

In the post-war period European investigators, including Lamy in France and Wiedemann in Germany, continued the process of delineation and their work has been carried further by Maroteaux in Paris and Spranger in Mainz. In the United States of America McKusick at the Johns Hopkins Hospital, Baltimore, made noteworthy contributions and many of his former pupils and colleagues are now active in this field. McKusick's catalogue of genetic disorders 'Mendelian Inheritance in Man', which reached its fifth edition in 1979, contains much information concerning the inherited skeletal dysplasias and plays an important role in their continuing elucidation. During the same era Rubin published his 'Dynamic Classification of Bone Dysplasias', in which these conditions were grouped according to the anatomical distribution of the skeletal changes, and many of Rubin's ideas have been incorporated into current concepts.

In the past decade a succession of Birth Defects meetings held in the United States, and sponsored by the 'March of Dimes' charity, has facilitated contact between investigators in the field of inherited bone dysplasias and catalysed the development of ideas and knowledge concerning these conditions.

3.3 Nomenclature

In the 1960s the explosion of interest in the inherited skeletal dysplasias promoted international contact and collaboration. Problems of communication arose since these rare conditions often had several names, some of which were eponyms, while others were descriptive or pertained to the underlying defect. Not infrequently each author who reported an additional case in the early literature employed a different designation for the disorder, and consequently semantic confusion became a major difficulty. This problem was eventually ameliorated in 1969 when the European Society of Paediatric Radiologists convened a meeting in Paris to attempt to unify existing terminology. The resulting 'International Nomenclature of Constitutional Disorders of Bone' was promulgated in 1970 and comprised a list of designations for approximately 200 conditions. These were grouped together in several categories, but the committee of experts emphasised that their intention was to produce an agreed nomenclature rather than a classification. Certain general principles were followed, such as the avoidance of eponyms or cumbersome names, and the Paris Nomenclature has subsequently proved to be an effective basis for communication and the publication of information.

This group re-convened in Paris in 1977 to bring the Nomenclature up to date. A few disorders were added or deleted and established heterogeneity was indicated. The word 'dysplasia' was substituted for 'dwarfism' in the titles of all conditions in which it appeared, since it was felt that the latter term might prove offensive. The new version of the Paris Nomenclature, which was published in 1978, is given below:

International Nomenclature of Constitutional Disease of Bone

Osteochondrodysplasias
Abnormalities of cartilage and/or bone growth and development.

Defects of growth of tubular bones and/or spine
A. Identifiable at birth
 1. Achondrogenesis type I, Parenti-Fraccaro
 2. Achondrogenesis type II, Langer-Saldino
 3. Thanatophoric dysplasia

 4. Thanatophoric dysplasia with clover-leaf skull
 5. Short rib-polydactyly syndrome type I, Saldino-Noonan (perhaps several forms)
 6. Short rib-polydactyly syndrome type II, Majewski
 7. Chondrodysplasia punctata
 a. Rhizomelic form

b. Dominant form
c. Other forms, excluding symptomatic stippling in other disorders (e.g., Zellweger syndrome, Warfarin embryopathy)
8. Campomelic dysplasia
9. Other dysplasias with congenital bowing of long bones (several forms)
10. Achondroplasia
11. Diastrophic dysplasia
12. Metatropic dysplasia (several forms)
13. Chondroectodermal dysplasia, Ellis Van Creveld
14. Asphyxiating thoracic dysplasia, Jeune
15. Spondyloepiphyseal dysplasia congenita
    a. Type Spranger-Wiedemann
    b. Other forms (see B, 11–12)
16. Kniest dysplasia
17. Mesomelic dysplasia
    a. Type Nievergelt
    b. Type Langer (probable homozygous dyschondrosteosis)
    c. Type Robinow
    d. Type Rheinhardt
    e. Other forms
18. Acromesomelic dysplasia
19. Cleidocranial dysplasia
20. Larsen syndrome
21. Otopalatodigital syndrome
B. Identifiable in later life
1. Hypochondroplasia
2. Dyschondrosteosis
3. Metaphyseal chondrodysplasia type Jansen
4. Metaphyseal chondrodysplasia type Schmid
5. Metaphyseal chondrodysplasia type McKusick.
6. Metaphyseal chondrodysplasia with exocrine pancreatic insufficiency and cyclic neutropenia
7. Spondylometaphyseal dysplasia
    a. Type Kozlowski
    b. Other forms
8. Multiple epiphyseal dysplasia
    a. Type Fairbank
    b. Other forms
9. Arthro-opthalmopathy, Stickler
10. Pseudoachondroplasia
    a. Dominant
    b. Recessive
11. Spondyloepiphyseal dysplasia tarda
12. Spondyloepiphyseal dysplasia, other forms (see A, 15–16)
13. Dyggve-Melchior-Clausen dysplasia
14. Spondyloepimetaphyseal dysplasia (several forms)
15. Myotonic chondrodysplasia, Catel-Schwartz-Jampel
16. Parastremmatic dysplasia
17. Trichorhinophalangeal dysplasia
18. Acrodysplasia with retinitis pigmentosa and nephropathy Saldino-Mainzer

Disorganized development of cartilage and fibrous components of skeleton
1. Dysplasia epiphysealis hemimelica
2. Multiple cartilaginous exostoses
3. Acrodysplasia with exostoses, Giedion-Langer
4. Enchondromatosis, Ollier
5. Enchondromatosis with hemangioma, Maffucci
6. Metachondromatosis
7. Fibrous dysplasia, Jaffe-Lichtenstein
8. Fibrous dysplasia with skin pigmentation and precocious puberty, McCune-Albright
9. Cherubism (familial fibrous dysplasia of the jaws)
10. Neurofibromatosis

Abnormalities of density of cortical diaphyseal structure and/or metaphyseal modelling
1. Osteogenesis imperfecta congenita (several forms)
2. Osteogenesis imperfecta tarda (several forms)
3. Juvenile idiopathic osteoporosis
4. Osteoporosis with pseudoglioma
5. Osteopetrosis with precocious manifestations
6. Osteopetrosis with delayed manifestations (several forms)
7. Pycnodysostosis
8. Osteopoikilosis
9. Osteopathia striata
10. Melorheostosis
11. Diaphyseal dysplasia, Camurati-Engelmann
12. Craniodiaphyseal dysplasia
13. Endosteal hyperostosis
    a. Autosomal dominant, Worth
    b. Autosomal recessive, Van Buchem
14. Tubular stenosis, Kenny-Caffey
15. Pachydermoperiostosis
16. Osteodysplasty, Melnick-Needles
17. Frontometaphyseal dysplasia
18. Craniometaphyseal dysplasia (several forms)
19. Metaphyseal dysplasia, Pyle
20. Sclerosteosis
21. Dysosteosclerosis
22. Osteoectasia with hyperphosphatasia

Dysostoses
Malformation of individual bones singly or in combination.

Dysostoses with cranial and facial involvement
1. Craniosynostosis (several forms)
2. Craniofacial dysostosis, Crouzon
3. Acrocephalosyndactyly, Apert (and others)
4. Acrocephalopolysyndactyly, Carpenter (and others)
5. Mandibulofacial dysostosis
    a. Type Treacher Collins, Franceschetti

b. Other forms
6. Oculomandibulofacial syndrome, Haller-mann-Streiff-Francois
7. Nevoid basal cell carcinoma syndrome

Dysostoses with predominant axial involvement
1. Vertebral segmentation defects, including Klippel-Feil
2. Cervico-oculoacoustic syndrome, Wilder-vanck
3. Sprengel anomaly
4. Spondylocostal dysostosis
   a. Dominant form
   b. Recessive forms
5. Oculovertebral syndrome, Weyers
6. Osteo-onychodysostosis
7. Cerebrocostomandibular syndrome

Dysostoses with predominant involvement of extremities
1. Acheiria
2. Apodia
3. Ectrodactyly syndrome
4. Aglossia-adactyly syndrome
5. Congenital bowing of long bones (several forms) (see also osteochondrodysplasias)
6. Familial radioulnar synostosis
7. Brachydactyly (several forms)
8. Symphalangism
9. Polydactyly (several forms)
10. Syndactyly (several forms)
11. Polysyndactyly (several forms)
12. Camptodactyly
13. Poland syndrome
14. Rubinstein-Taybi syndrome
15. Pancytopenia-dysmelia syndrome, Fanconi
16. Thrombocytopenia-radialaplasia syndrome
17. Orodigitofacial syndrome
    a. Type Papillon-Leage
    b. Type Mohr
18. Cardiomelic syndrome, Holt-Oram (and others)
19. Femoral facial syndrome
20. Multiple synostoses (includes some forms of symphalangism)
21. Scapuloiliac dysostosis, Kosenow-Sinios
22. Hand-foot-genital syndrome
23. Focal dermal hypoplasia, Goltz

Idiopathic Osteolyses
1. Phalangeal (several forms)
2. Tarsocarpal
   a. Including Francois form (and others)
   b. With nephropathy
3. Multicentric
   a. Hajdu-Cheney form
   b. Winchester form
   c. Other forms

Chromosomal Aberrations
Specific entities not listed

Primary Metabolic Abnormalities
Calcium and/or phosphorus
1. Hypophosphatemic rickets
2. Pseudodeficiency rickets, Prader, Royer
3. Late rickets, McCance
4. Idiopathic hypercalcuria
5. Hypophosphatasia (several forms)
6. Pseudohypoparathyroidism (normo- and hypo-calcaemic forms, include acrodysostosis)

Complex carbohydrates
1. Mucopolysaccharidosis, type I (alpha-L-iduronidase deficiency)
   a. Hurler form
   b. Scheie form
   c. Other forms
2. Mucopolysaccharidosis, type II, Hunter (sulfoiduronate sulfatase deficiency)
3. Mucopolysaccharidosis, type III San Filippo
   a. Type A (heparin sulfamidase deficiency)
   b. Type B (N-acetyl-alpha-glucosamini-dase deficiency)
4. Mucopolysaccharidosis, type IV, Morquio (N-acetylgalactosamine-6-sulfate-sulfatase deficiency)
5. Mucopolysaccharidosis, type VI, Maroteaux-Lamy (aryl sulfatase B deficiency)
6. Mucopolysaccharidosis, type VII (beta-glucuronidase deficiency)
7. Aspartylglucosaminuria (aspartyl-glucosaminidase deficiency)
8. Mannosidosis (alpha-mannosidase deficiency)
9. Fucosidosis (alpha-fucosidase deficiency)
10. GMI-gangliosidosis (beta-galactosidase deficiency)
11. Multiple sulfatase deficiency, Austin, Thieffry
12. Neuraminidase deficiency (formerly muco-lipidosis I)
13. Mucolipidosis II
14. Mucolipidosis III

Lipids
1. Niemann-Pick disease
2. Gaucher disease

Nucleic acids
1. Adenosine-deaminase deficiency and others

Amino acids
1. Homocystinuria and others

Metals
1. Menkes kinky hair syndrome and others

3.4 Classification

Apart from Rubin's classification of dysplasias on strictly anatomical criteria most methods of categorisation have been rather tentative. The simple format adopted in this book has been chosen to provide a convenient framework for division into chapters. Although the contents of most chapters fit satisfactorily into their descriptive niche, the number of entities grouped in Chapter 15 under the heading of 'Miscellaneous Disorders' will indicate the extent of the difficulties encountered in attempting a comprehensive classification.

3.5 Terminology

A number of terms which are in general use in the context of inherited skeletal dysplasias warrant consideration. For example, 'dwarfism' has the connotation of reduced height, but there is no absolute definition of this attribute, as ethnic and constitutional factors interact with the fundamental genetic abnormality in the determination of stature. Therefore a person's height can only be considered abnormal in relation to that of his normal peers. Thus the normal stature of the Kalahari Bushmen would meet the North American criteria for dwarfism. In general usage 'dwarfism' implies a pathological diminution in height, whereas 'short stature' denotes height which is at the lower end of the normal range for the population under consideration.

Dwarfism is conventionally regarded as being proportionate or disproportionate and the latter category is subdivided into short-limbed and short-trunked forms. The non-medical term 'midget' is sometimes used to denote proportionate dwarfism, while short-limbed dwarfs may be further sub-categorised on an anatomical basis into rhizomelic, mesomelic, and acromelic varieties. These terms indicate that shortening is maximal in the proximal, middle, or distal portions of the limbs, respectively. The term 'dysplasia' implies generalised skeletal change, whereas 'dysosotosis' denotes involvement of a single bone or segment. 'Malformation' indicates a primary abnormality of development, while 'deformity' describes a structure which was previously normal but has undergone modification.

3.6 Current Trends

Delineation of rare syndromes is largely dependent upon the accumulation of adequate clinical, radiographic, and genetic data. In the past this was a gradual process, as with the Fairbank collection, but the formation of organisations which cater for the special needs of persons with specific skeletal problems has enabled more rapid accumulation of information. The aim of these societies is to provide contact and support on a basis that 'problems shared are problems halved'. They also provide links with medical and para-medical services and act as pressure groups at a socio-political level.

Perhaps the best-known is the 'Little People of America' which caters for persons of short stature and has several thousand members. In the same way, the 'Brittle Bone Society' is concerned with osteogenesis imperfecta and related disorders. In recent years similar groups have been established in many parts of the world. The majority of such organisations are interested in medical research and therefore comparatively large numbers of persons with rare disorders are available for investigation.

The development of skeletal dysplasia registers has provided a similar opportunity for the accumulation and analysis of clinical and radiographic material. This information can now be recorded in computers and it is likely that international links between such data banks will be established. This will give further impetus to the process of syndrome delineation.

4. Disorders of Epiphyses and Metaphyses with Predominant Epiphyseal Involvement

The epiphyses of the tubular bones are principally affected in a number of inherited skeletal dysplasias, while the remainder of the skeleton is relatively normal.

Multiple epiphyseal dysplasia (M.E.D.) is by far the most common of these, but the various forms of chondrodysplasia punctata also warrant consideration by virtue of their important complications. The hereditary basis of dysplasia epiphysealis hemimelica is uncertain, but the epiphyseal changes warrant its inclusion in this chapter.

4.1 Multiple Epiphyseal Dysplasia

There are numerous varieties of M.E.D., including a mild 'Ribbing' and a more severe 'Fairbank' type. The wide overlap in clinical and radiological appearances between recognised categories may make precise delineation difficult.

Clinical Features

Moderate short stature and 'knobbly' joints may be noticed in childhood. The digits are stubby in some forms of M.E.D., and mild spinal involvement sometimes occurs which may result in short stature. Children may have difficulty in walking or running but there is often surprisingly little disability, and the early onset of pain in the weight-bearing joints may be the first indication of the disease. A skeletal survey and a positive family history might then suggest the diagnosis. The life expectancy and intelligence are normal.

Radiographic Appearances (Figs. 4.1–4.3)

The epiphyses of the long bones appear late and present an irregular, mottled, flattened appearance. When the hands are affected, ossification of the carpal centres is delayed and the epiphyses of the digits are all involved. The femoral capital epiphyses are nearly always abnormal, producing flattened, misshapen femoral heads, but the acetabulae are not primarily affected. In adulthood the appearances of the joints may be surprisingly normal, but valgus or varus deformity of the knees may occur and early degenerative changes commonly develop in the hips and knees. The vertebrae are normal or show only mild platyspondyly and irregularity of the end-plates.

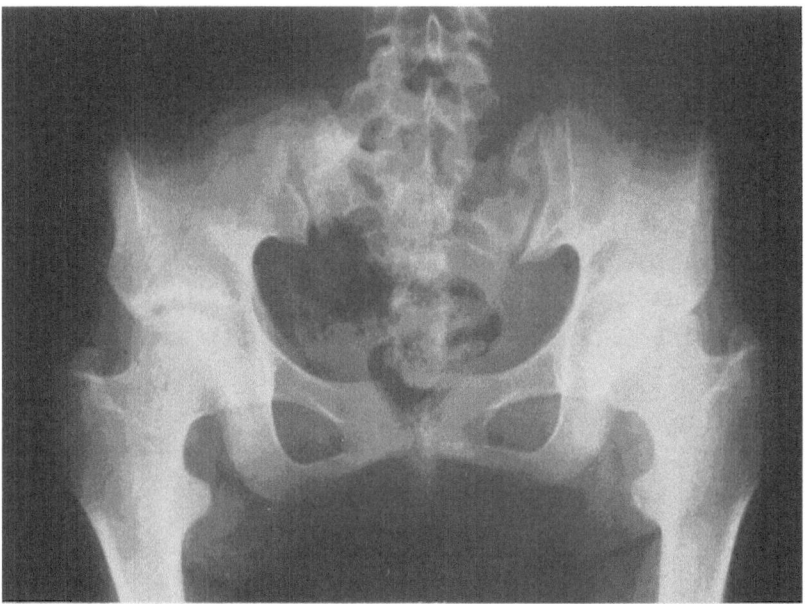

Fig. 4.1. Multiple epiphyseal dysplasia. AP view of the pelvis shows irregularity of the femoral capital epiphyses with a normal acetabulum.

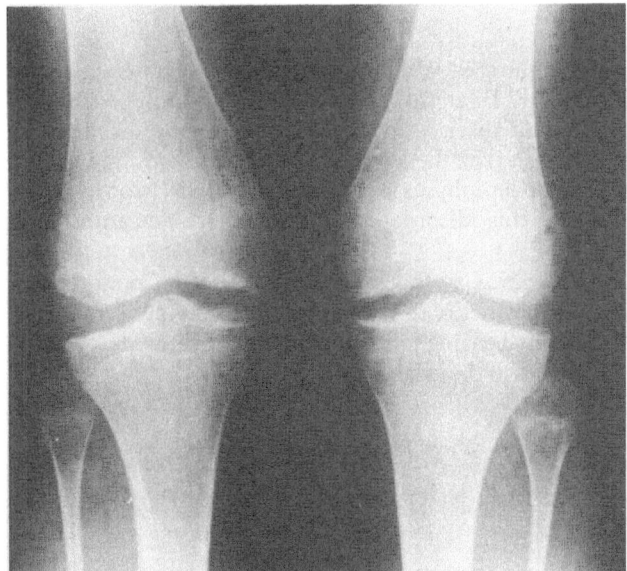

Fig. 4.2. Multiple epiphyseal dysplasia. The knees show epiphyseal irregularity.

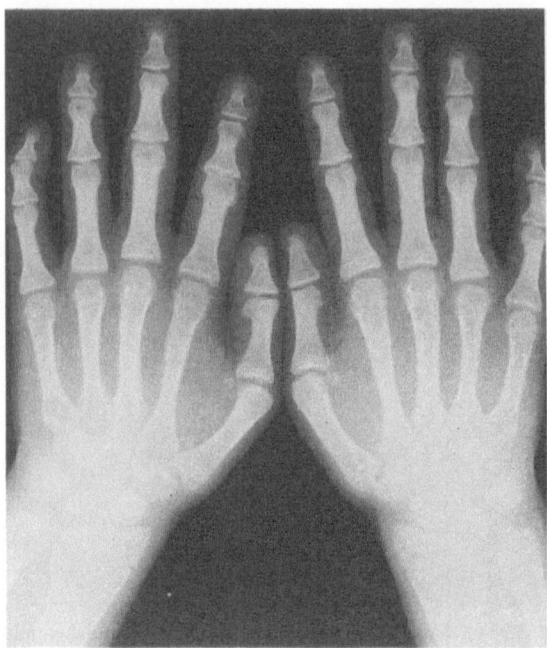

Fig. 4.3. Multiple epiphyseal dysplasia. The wrists and hands show widespread epiphyseal abnormality.

Genetics

Multiple epiphyseal dysplasia is extremely heterogeneous but it is usually inherited as an autosomal dominant trait.

Management

Problems in childhood are rarely encountered, although walking may be delayed and mild joint stiffness can be troublesome. Bilateral involvement of the upper femoral epiphyses may be mistaken for Perthes' disease and a skeletal survey must then be undertaken before this latter diagnosis can be confidently established. However, familial dysplasia of the upper femoral epiphyses has been described (Monty 1962; Wamoscher and Farhi 1963), and this disorder is inherited as an autosomal dominant.

In early adulthood, residual deformity at the knee may cause discomfort and corrective osteotomy is indicated for cosmetic, functional and prophylactic reasons. Onset of pain and stiffness in the weight-bearing joints may be surprisingly late, but if severe symptoms develop replacement arthroplasty will be required.

4.2 Chondrodysplasia Punctata (Stippled Epiphyses)

Stippling of the epiphyses occurs in a variety of conditions including multiple epiphyseal dysplasia, spondylo-epiphyseal dysplasia, hypothyroidism, trisomy 18, trisomy 21 and the foetal warfarin syndrome (Silverman 1961; Pauli et al. 1976). The term 'stippled epiphyses' is also used as an alternative name for chondrodysplasia punctata, which has two principal forms.

4.2.1 Conradi-Hünerman Type

Clinical Features

Infants have a flat face with a depressed nasal bridge, and atrophic skin changes and congenital cataracts may be seen. Asymmetric shortening of the limbs and a scoliosis, which can be rapidly progressive, are the most important orthopaedic complications. Joint contractures may develop and vary in their site and severity. Severely affected children may be stillborn but the majority survive to a normal life span. Moderate shortness of stature may be the only manifestation of the disorder in later childhood.

Radiographic Appearances (Fig. 4.4)

Punctate calcification is present in the epiphyses of the long bones, vertebrae and pelvis in infancy but usually disappears by the age of four (Tasker et al. 1970). Epiphyseal changes subsequently develop at the site of the 'stippling'. Asymmetrical shortening of the long bones is sometimes seen while irregular malformation of the vertebral bodies may produce scoliosis.

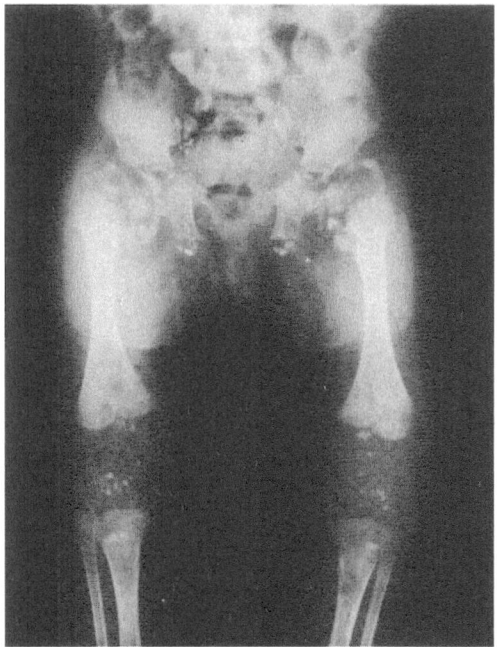

Fig. 4.4. Chondrodysplasia punctata, Conradi-Hünerman type. Multiple epiphyseal stippling is evident in the lower limbs, spine and pelvis. From Heselson et al. 1978.

Genetics

The condition is heterogeneous but the most common forms are inherited as autosomal dominant traits.

Management

Joint contractures, inequality of limb length and scoliosis are the principal skeletal problems. The severity of an individual contracture may vary and consequently definitive treatment should be delayed as long as possible. Shortness of a leg is best treated by operation for arrest of the appropriate epiphyses on the opposite side, since there is a high incidence of non-union when lengthening of the tibia or femur is attempted. Mild scoliosis can be managed by observation or, if more severe, by external bracing, but deterioration may be rapid and correction and fusion is then necessary.

4.2.2 Rhizomelic Form

Clinical Features

The majority of these infants are stillborn or die in the first year of life. They have marked proximal limb shortening as well as the facial, ocular, and dermal abnormalities which are found in the other forms of chondrodysplasia punctata. Joint contractures may occur and can cause dislocation at the hip.

Radiographic Appearances

In contrast to the Conradi-Hunerman form the lesions are symmetrical, with severe proximal limb shortening and mild metaphyseal widening. Extra-cartilaginous stippling is present, often in relation to the vertebral bodies. The dorsal and ventral ossification centres in the vertebral bodies are separated by a clear cartilaginous bar, which gives the appearance of a coronal cleft.

Genetics

Genetic transmission is autosomal recessive.

Management

In view of the poor prognosis, active orthopaedic intervention is unwarranted.

4.3 Dysplasia Epiphysealis Hemimelica

Dysplasia epiphysealis hemimelica is a disorder of unknown aetiology in which eccentric overgrowth of one side of an epiphysis occurs. The condition was described by Trevor (1950) who termed it 'tarso-epiphyseal aclasis' while Fairbank (1956) coined the current name.

Clinical Features

Pain, swelling and limitation of movement develop at the affected joint without any constitutional disturbance. The lower limb is involved most frequently with the distal tibia, talus and knee being the common sites, while lesions are sometimes seen in the carpal epiphyses. The onset of symptoms usually commences in early childhood but presentation may be delayed until puberty, and the occasional patient has first been seen well into adulthood (Kettelkamp et al. 1966). These authors, in a detailed review, reported multiple lesions on the same side of a single limb in two-thirds of cases, and stated that males were affected three times more frequently than females.

Radiographic Appearances (Fig. 4.5)

One side of the affected epiphysis shows enlargement and irregularity, which may appear to be detached from the main epiphysis and have additional small areas of ossification. If the tarsus is involved the outgrowth may be large, nodulated and irregular. Wolfgang and Heath (1976) described a child with widespread involvement of the lateral side of the ankle and hindfoot, while Buckwater et al. (1978) described mild deformity of the forearm and carpus in a boy whose distal ulnar epiphysis was affected.

Management

Histologically the lesion is an osteochondroma. Removal of the outgrowth is indicated if it is producing symptoms, mechanical problems or deformity, since the remainder of the epiphysis will then often grow normally. Leg length discrepancy may arise and is managed by epiphysiodesis if necessary.

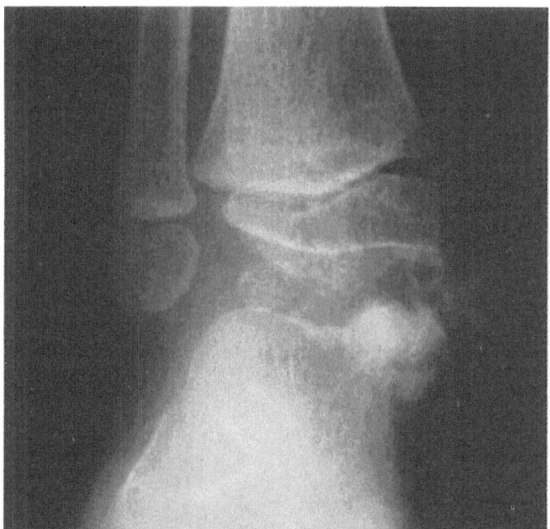

Fig. 4.5. Dysplasia epiphysealis hemimelica. A large, nodular outgrowth is associated with the medial side of the lower tibial epiphysis.

References

Multiple Epiphyseal Dysplasia

Monty CP (1962) Familial Perthes' disease resembling multiple epiphyseal dysplasia. J Bone Joint Surg [Br] 44:565
Wamoscher Z, Farhi A (1963) Hereditary Legg-Calve-Perthes' disease. Am J Dis Child 106:131

Chondrodysplasia Punctata

Heselson NG, Cremin BJ, Beighton PH (1978) Lethal chondrodysplasia punctata. Clin Radiol 29:679
Pauli MP, Madden JD, Kranzler KJ, Culpeper W, Port R (1970) Warfarin therapy initiated during pregnancy and phenotypic chondrodysplasia punctata. J Pediatr 88:506
Silverman FN (1961) Dysplasie epiphysaires: entités protéiformes. Ann Radiol 4:833
Tasker WG, Mastri AR, Gold AP (1970) Chondrodystrophia calcificans congenita (dysplasia epiphysialis punctata). Recognition of the clinical picture. Am J Dis Child, 119:122

Dysplasia Epiphysealis Hemimelica

Fairbank TJ (1956) Dysplasia epiphysealis hemimelica (tarso-epiphyseal aclasis). J Bone Joint Surg [Br] 28:237
Kettelkamp DB, Campbell CJ, Bonfiglio M (1966) Dysplasia epiphysealis hemimelica. J Bone Joint Surg [Am] 48:746
Trevor D (1950) Tarso-epiphyseal aclasis: a congenital error of epiphyseal development. J Bone Joint Surg [Br] 32:204
Wolfgang GL, Heath RD (1976) Dysplasia epiphysealis hemimelica. A case report. Clin Orthop 116:23

5. Disorders of the Epiphyses and Metaphyses with Predominant Metaphyseal Involvement

The most important disorders in this category are achondroplasia, hypochondroplasia and the metaphyseal dysplasias. The spine and epiphyses may be involved to some degree in each, but metaphyseal changes predominate.

5.1 Achondroplasia

Achondroplasia is by far the commonest form of dwarfism and achondroplasts have been depicted in paintings and sculptures since ancient times. In the past, the term 'achondroplast' has been indiscriminately applied to any form of short-limbed dwarfism, but its use is now restricted to the specific entity described in this section.

Clinical Features (Fig. 5.1)

The limbs are disproportionately short, with the proximal segment particularly affected. The forehead is prominent and the nasal bridge depressed. The fingers are short and stubby and inability to approximate the extended fingers produces a characteristic 'trident' appearance of the hand. Achondroplasts are usually of normal mentality, but hydrocephalus is present in a few. Delay in acquiring motor skills due to the underlying skeletal dysplasia may give an inaccurate indication of mental retardation. Walking is usually delayed until about 20 months, after which the protuberant abdomen, prominent buttocks, and hip flexion contractures become apparent. A marked lumbar lordosis is seen when standing and bilateral genu varum may produce bowing of the legs. Full extension of the elbow cannot be achieved and supination of the forearms may be limited.

A mid-spinal kyphosis may develop in infancy, but usually disappears after walking has commenced. If this deformity persists into later life the risk of developing cord compression is seriously increased. Genu varum develops during late childhood and valgus deformity of the foot may be established by the end of adolescence. Apart from the lumbar lordosis, about 70% of achondroplasts develop some degree of spinal malalignment (Bailey 1970), with 40% experiencing neurological disturbance (Kopits 1972).

Radiographic Appearances (Figs. 5.2 and 5.3)

The calvarium is large, with prominence of the frontal, parietal, and occipital regions and apparent shortening of the base of the skull. The foramen magnum is smaller than normal. The interpedicular distance diminishes from the upper to the lower lumbar spine, and the pedicles are short, reducing the anteroposterior diameter of the spinal canal. The appearance of the pelvis is characteristic, with squared iliac wings, a horizontal lower margin of the ilium and a small greater sciatic notch. The limb bones are short with wide metaphyses which may show mild irregularity. The epiphyses are relatively normal. Coxa valga and genu varum may be evident.

Genetics

Inheritance is autosomal dominant and the clinical expression is consistent. About 80% of achondroplasts are examples of gene mutation and have normal parents.

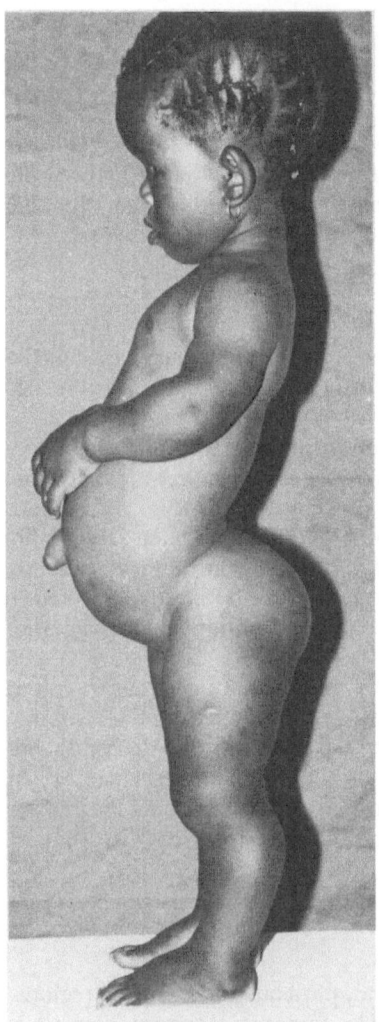

Fig. 5.1. Achondroplasia in a child. Frontal bossing, a depressed nasal bridge, prominence of the abdomen and buttocks, lumbar lordosis and proximal limb shortening are the major clinical features.

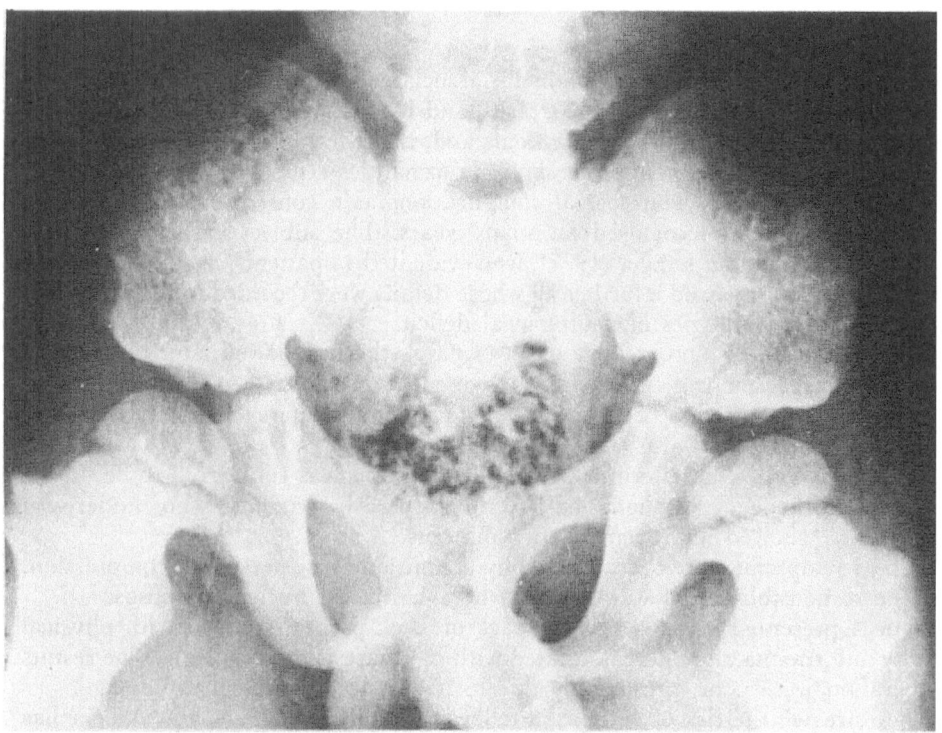

Fig. 5.2. Antero-posterior view of the pelvis of an adolescent achondroplast. The iliac wings are square, the greater sciatic notch is small and the upper femoral metaphyses are flared; the epiphyses are normal.

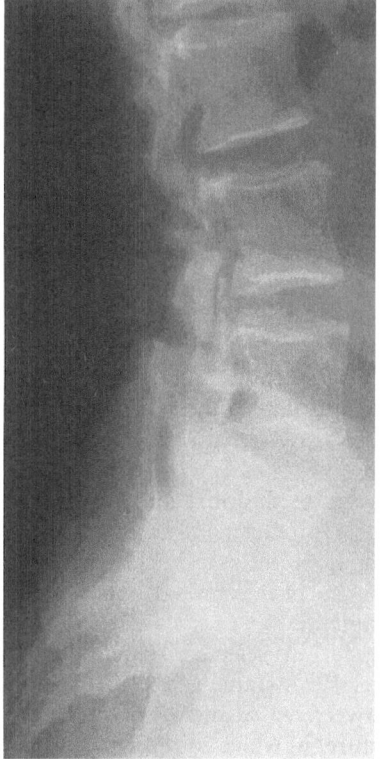

Fig. 5.3. Lateral view of the lumbosacral spine in an adult with achondroplasia showing the short pedicles and flattened lumbar canal.

Management

The management of the skeletal problems associated with achondroplasia has been extensively reviewed by Bailey (1970, 1973) and Kopits (1976). The back and lower limbs are the principal source of problems and, apart from recurrent ear infections and occasional hydrocephalus, the skull abnormalities seldom present difficulty.

The development of neurological complications as a consequence of the spinal deformities has been recognised for many years. The subject has recently been reviewed by Lutter and Langer (1977), who evaluated 14 patients on whom they had carried out operations and a further 29 whose details were recorded in the literature. They described four types of neurological deficit.

Type 1 had a slow, progressive onset of paraesthesia followed later by sensory, motor and reflex changes. It was most frequently associated with thoraco-lumbar kyphosis, and appeared to be due to mechanical compression of the cord. Improvement after laminectomy was unpredictable.

Type 2 involved true intermittent claudication and was considered to be due to vascular insufficiency brought on by activity. All patients who underwent laminectomy showed improvement in symptoms.

Type 3 symptoms were characterised by the onset of true nerve root compression, and the responsible lesion was found to be a herniated nucleus pulposus.

Type 4 presented as acute, severe back or neck pain, associated with physical activity and trauma and often associated with paraparesis or paraplegia. The results of operation were poor, presumably due to irreversible neurological damage.

They stressed the risk of paraplegia following laminectomy, and this danger has also been recognised by Nelson (1980, personal communication). Lutter et al. (1977) drew attention to the thickness of the pedicles and inferior facets in the lumbar spine in achondroplasia, and emphasised the need for adequate foraminotomy when decompression was undertaken. They suggested that subsequent instability might require spinal fusion, but in nine patients mentioned by Kopits (1976) who had undergone extensive decompression, fusion had not been necessary. Kopitz also noted that cord compression sometimes occurred at the foramen magnum, which may have an abnormally small diameter in some patients. Morgan and Young (1980) classified spinal stenosis in achondroplasia according to the affected level in 17 patients. Ten patients had compression at the thoracolumbar level and five at the upper cervical spine or foramen magnum, while two had generalised stenosis. Decompression gave excellent results in the first two groups but the third group progressively deteriorated despite operation.

The weight-bearing joints are surprisingly free from trouble and degenerative changes are encountered infrequently. When indicated the tibia vara can be corrected by osteotomy, and a modified opening wedge has been advocated. The method of osteotomy/osteoclasis may also be employed.

Valgus deformity of the foot is secondary to bowing of the tibia and may give problems due to pain or difficulty with shoe fitting. Impingement of the lateral malleolus against the calcaneum may occur if the hindfoot lies in valgus, when the fibula appears overlong. Supramalleolar osteotomy by one of the methods mentioned above can be used to achieve a satisfactory realignment.

Attempts at leg lengthening may prove successful in selected patients and significant gains in height have been achieved (Pfluger 1977; Ganel et al. 1979). The latter authors achieved a gain in leg length of between 33% and 44% in three achondroplasts by repeated use of the Wagner procedure, in which initial distraction was achieved by an outrigger appliance after which the bone was stabilised by a plate and a bone graft applied. Two children had their first operation at the age of $3\frac{1}{2}$ years and the authors suggested that the procedures should be carried out between growth spurts. The potential complications of such operations are considerable and infection, transient nerve paralysis and refracture were encountered.

5.2 Hypochondroplasia

Hypochondroplasia is probably relatively common, but as it is clinically innocuous, many affected persons remain undiagnosed or unreported and the true frequency is unknown. At the clinical and radiographic level the condition is best regarded as a mild form of achondroplasia, but genetically these conditions are separate and distinct and there is no intra-familial overlap.

Clinical Features

Hypochondroplasia resembles achondroplasia in that there is short stature with mild rhizomelia, but the stigmata are much less obvious and the skull, face, and fingers are virtually unaffected. The condition becomes apparent in early childhood, when skeletal disproportion, a mild lumbar lordosis, limitation of full extension of the elbow joints, and genu varum may be seen. Moderate generalised joint laxity has been described (Beals 1969). The severity of the clinical features is variable and the appearance may be almost normal. About 20% of hypochondroplasts are mentally subnormal.

Radiographic Appearances (Fig. 5.4)

The skull and hands are not usually involved, although occasionally the cranium may be slightly enlarged. The vertebral canal is narrowed in the antero-posterior projection and the interpedicular distances may be diminished in the lumbar spine, although not as much as in achondroplasia. The sacrum is hypoplastic and tends to lie horizontally with respect to the lower lumbar vertebrae. The femoral necks are small and short with a normal neck/shaft angle, but the femoral capital epiphyses may lie in slight varus. The tubular bones are short and broadened, whilst the distal portion of the fibula may be overlong in relation to the tibia and result in a varus deformity of the hindfoot. The radiographic changes in some persons are of minor degree and the diagnosis is not always easily made.

Genetics

Hypochondroplasia is usually inherited as an autosomal dominant, but the presence of mental retardation in some individuals may indicate heterogeneity.

Management

Orthopaedic complications are uncommon and no specific measures are indicated. It is of passing interest that hypochondroplasts have been successful in the spheres of Olympic weight lifting and international rugby, in which their powerful build in relation to their short stature might be advantageous. Musculoskeletal injuries sustained in these activities have healed in a normal manner with standard treatment.

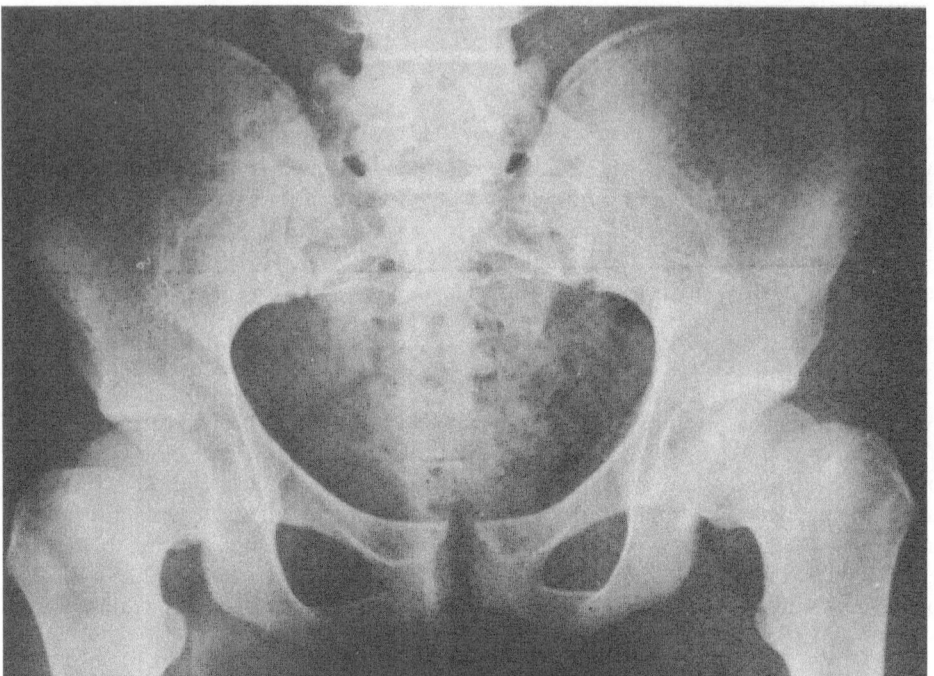

Fig. 5.4. Hypochondroplasia. The femoral necks are short and the epiphyses have closed in slight varus. The interpedicular distances of the lower lumbar vertebrae are narrow. From Heselson et al. 1979.

5.3 Metaphyseal Chondrodysplasia

The metaphyseal chondrodysplasias are a group of uncommon disorders in which the principal abnormality resides in the metaphyses of the long bones. An attempt at a comprehensive description of these disorders is outside the scope of this book and only the better known syndromes will be considered.

5.3.1 Metaphyseal Chondrodysplasia: Schmid Type

Clinical Features

This is the commonest of the metaphyseal chondrodysplasias. Mild to moderate short stature and bowing of the legs are apparent in early childhood and these features remain in the mature adult. Bilateral coxa vara is usually present and may lead to a waddling gait. The lumbar spine is lordotic but other spinal abnormalities are infrequent.

Radiographic Appearances (Fig. 5.5)

The metaphyses of the long bones are splayed and irregular and may be cupped, presenting an appearance resembling healing rickets. In childhood the changes are most marked at the knees, particularly on the medial side of the metaphyses, but later the most striking appearance may be in the femoral neck, where the metaphyseal abnormality results in a coxa vara deformity. The epiphyses are normal.

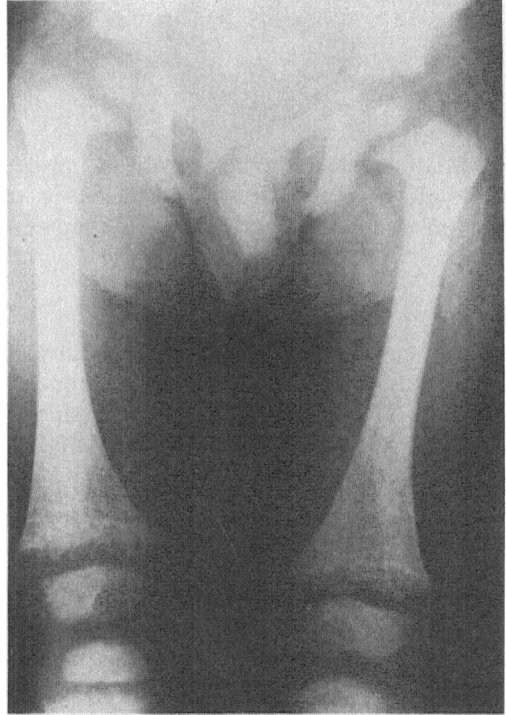

Fig. 5.5. Metaphyseal chondroplasia, Schmid type. The metaphyses are splayed and capped. The epiphyses are normal. The metaphyseal abnormality has produced a coxa vara.

Genetics

The Schmid form of metaphyseal chondrodysplasia is inherited as an autosomal dominant with marked variation of expression.

Management

Coxa vara and bow legs present the principal problems. During childhood, development of significant coxa vara warrants subtrochanteric valgus osteotomy to improve gait and to gain a little height, and pain in the knees may require upper tibial osteotomy to correct the varus deformity (Wasylenko et al. 1980). This operation may be necessary in the adult to stabilise the mechanics of weight-bearing. Differentiation from dietary or metabolic rickets is sometimes difficult although the biochemical abnormalities found in these disorders are not present in the metaphyseal chondrodysplasia of Schmid. Recurrence of the deformity following corrective osteotomy indicates that the diagnosis warrants reappraisal. Blount disease may also be confused with the metaphyseal chondrodysplasias, but in this disorder the radiographic changes are confined to the region of the knee joint, with involvement principally of the medial portions of the upper tibial epiphysis and metaphysis.

It has been observed by several authors (Dent and Normand 1958; Evans and Caffey 1958; Wasylenko et al. 1980) that the radiographic abnormalities observed at the metaphyseal growth plate revert to normal after prolonged immobilisation, but rapidly reappear after weight-bearing begins again, suggesting that this region may have an abnormal response to stress.

5.3.2 Metaphyseal Chondrodysplasia: Jansen Type

This rare form of metaphyseal chondrodysplasia was the first to be described (Jansen 1934), and only a few cases have subsequently been reported. Nevertheless it is comparatively well known and is therefore given a brief mention in this chapter.

Clinical Features

Dwarfing becomes obvious in early infancy, with bowing of the lower limbs and arms. The joints are knobbly due to metaphyseal expansion and the feet may be clubbed. Involvement of the metacarpals and phalanges produces stubby, gnarled hands. Deafness may be a problem in adulthood. A raised level of serum calcium has been consistently found but symptoms of hypercalcaemia do not occur.

Radiographic Appearances

The most marked abnormalities are present in the metaphyses of the long bones which are expanded and have an irregular growth plate. Lucent areas of uncalcified cartilage lie adjacent to the growth plate, and the expanding metaphyses contain patches of calcification. The epiphyses and diaphyses are normal.

Genetics

All reported cases have been sporadic, except for a single instance of an affected mother and daughter. Inheritance is presumed to be autosomal dominant but remains unproven.

Management

Jansen's original patient has been followed up by de Haas et al. (1969) who reported few problems apart from dwarfism and deafness.

5.3.3 Metaphyseal Chondrodysplasia: McKusick Type

This condition was originally termed cartilage-hair hypoplasia and has been extensively studied by McKusick (1965) among the Amish, an inbred religious isolate living in Pennsylvania.

Clinical Features

These patients have short-limb dwarfism of varying degree with fine, sparse hair, eyebrows, and eyelashes. The hands and feet are short and stubby, and mild joint laxity is sometimes present, particularly in the hands.

Radiographic Appearances

The long bones are short with widening and irregularity of the metaphyses, which show cystic changes and patchy sclerosis across their entire extent. These abnormalities are most marked at the knee and at the upper end of the femur, where they vary from a 'ball in socket' configuration of the capital epiphysis on the metaphysis to an appearance which is suggestive of Perthes' disease with coxa vara (Beals 1968). The distal end of the fibula may be disproportionately long and an increase in vertebral body height has been noted.

Genetics

Inheritance is autosomal recessive.

Management

Associated medical problems include Hirchsprung disease and failure to thrive. Immunological competence is abnormal and severe reactions to varicella infection and smallpox vaccination may occur.

Orthopaedic complications are not unusually troublesome although avascular necrosis of the femoral head (Beals 1968) and persistent hindfoot varus may require operation.

5.3.4 Other Forms of Metaphyseal Chondrodysplasia

Several other types of metaphyseal chondrodysplasia have been delineated, but in view of their rarity further consideration in this chapter is not warranted. The reader will find detailed discussion of these entities in the major monographs which are listed in the Appendix.

5.4 Vitamin D-Resistant Rickets (Fig. 5.6)

Vitamin D-resistant rickets or familial hypophosphataemia is an inherited metabolic bone disease which presents in childhood with deformity of the lower limbs and may be confused with the metaphyseal chondrodysplasias. Rickets due to deficiency of diet and the rare forms which are secondary to genetic renal disease have similar manifestations, but their detailed consideration is outside the scope of this chapter.

Clinical Features

The lower limbs become bent when weight-bearing commences, with the development of bow legs, knock knees or a 'wind-swept' appearance with a valgus deformity

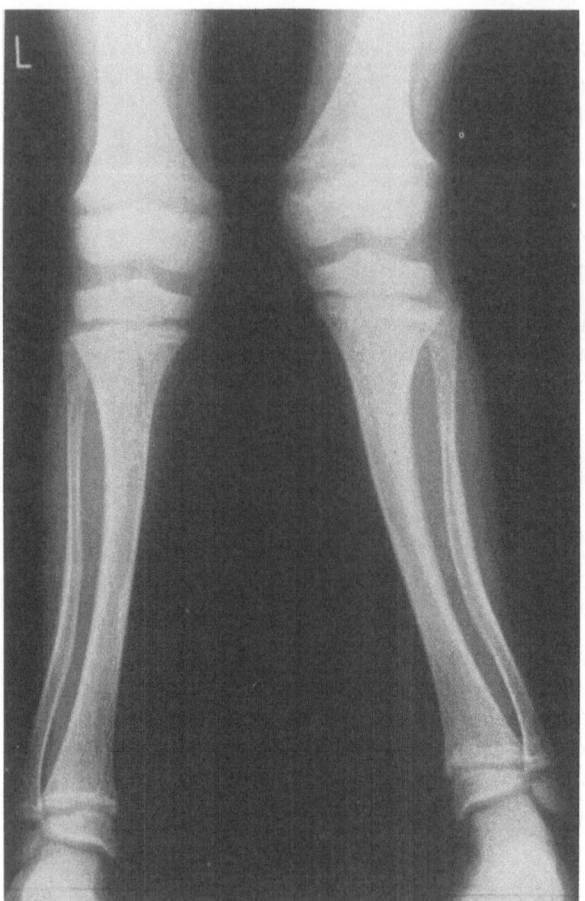

Fig. 5.6. Vitamin D-resistant rickets. Irregular, wide metaphyses, porosis, a coarse trabecular pattern, and cortical thinning are typical of rickets. This child has bilateral coxa valga but bowing of the legs is the usual deformity in this condition.

of one knee and a varus deformity of the other. The usual pattern seen is of lateral bowing of the tibia and fibula and anterolateral bowing of the femur. Expansion of the metaphyses may be obvious in all the long bones. The teeth may be abnormal and scoliosis develops in severe cases. Overall height may be reduced in adults, in whom bone pain and joint stiffness may prove troublesome.

The limb deformities are very variable in severity, and range from minimal changes to profound disablement. The condition is usually progressive throughout childhood but becomes static by the third decade and the general health is unimpaired.

Diagnosis is aided by the demonstration of a low serum phosphorus concentration, diminished absorption of phosphorus by the renal tubules and of calcium by the intestine, and by recognition of the typical pattern of inheritance.

Radiographic Appearances

In the active phase the metaphyses of all long bones are irregular and widened with the changes extending across the whole metaphysis, but the epiphyses are normal. The skeleton is porotic with cortical thinning and a coarse trabecular pattern, and pseudofractures or incomplete fractures may be present. Bowing of the long bones of the legs is usually seen. These appearances are indistinguishable from other forms of rickets.

Genetics

The classic form of vitamin D-resistant rickets is inherited as an X-linked dominant. In this unusual form of transmission all the daughters of an affected male would receive the faulty gene, whilst 50% of the sons of a mother with the condition would be affected.

Management

The medical treatment of hypophosphataemia is based upon massive dosage with vitamin D, but the management is complex and referral to a specialised metabolic unit is strongly recommended. Surgical correction of deformities of the lower limbs is advisable although recurrence is inevitable unless the disease has been brought under medical control. Recurrence may also suggest that an incorrect diagnosis has been made and a thorough metabolic investigation must then be instituted.

References

Achondroplasia

Bailey JA II (1970) Orthopaedic aspects of achondroplasia. J Bone Joint Surg [Am] 52:1285
Bailey JA II (1973) Disproportionate short stature. Saunders, Philadelphia London Toronto p 83
Ganel A, Horoszowski H, Kahmin M, Farine I (1979) Leg lengthening in achondroplastic children. Clin Orthop 144:194
Kopits SE (1976) Orthopaedic complications of dwarfism. Clin Orthop 114:153
Lutter LD, Langer LO (1977) Neurological complications in achondroplastic dwarfs–surgical treatment. J Bone Joint Surg [Am] 59:87
Lutter LD, Lonstein JE, Winter RB, Langer LO (1977) Anatomy of the achondroplastic lumbar canal. Clin Orthop 126:139
Morgan DF, Young RF (1980) Spinal neurological complications of achondroplasia. Results of surgical treatment. Neurosurgery 52:463
Pfluger W (1977) Leg lengthening in systemic skeletal disorders. Orthopaede 6:16

Hypochondroplasia

Beals RK (1969) Hypochondroplasia. J Bone Joint Surg. [Am] 51:728
Heselson NG, Cremin BJ, Beighton P (1979) The radiographic manifestations of hypochondroplasia. Clin Radiol 30:79

Metaphyseal Dysplasia: Schmid Type

Dent CE, Normand ICS (1958) Metaphyseal dysosotosis, type Schmid. Arch Dis Child 39:444

Evans R, Caffey J (1958) Metaphyseal dysostosis resembling Vitamin D-refractory rickets. Am J Dis Child 95:640

Wasylenko MJ, Wedge JH, Houston CS (1980) Metaphyseal chondrodysplasia, Schmid type. J Bone Joint Surg [Am] 62:660

Metaphyseal Chondrodysplasia (Jansen type)

de Haas WHD, de Boer W, Griffioen F (1969) Metaphyseal dysostosis. J Bone Joint Surg [Br] 51B:290

Jansen M (1934) Über atypische Chondrodystrophie (Achondroplasie) und über ein noch nicht beschriebene angeborene Wachsumstörung des Knochensystems: Metaphysäre Dysostosis. Orthop Chirurg 61:253

Metaphyseal Chondrodysplasia (McKusick type)

Beals RK (1968) Cartilage-hair hypoplasia: a case report. J Bone Joint Surg [Am] 50:1245

McKusick VA, Eldridge R, Hostetler JA, Ruangwir U, Egeland JA (1965) Dwarfism in the Amish: II cartilage-hair hypoplasia. Bull Johns Hopkins Hosp 116:285

6. Disorders of the Epiphyses and Metaphyses with Major Vertebral Involvement

Changes in the spine predominate in a number of inherited skeletal dysplasias which all share the feature of disproportionate short stature. In some spinal malalignment may lead to cardio-respiratory failure and paraplegia due to cord compression.

6.1 Spondyloepiphyseal Dysplasia (S.E.D.)

The spondyloepiphyseal dysplasias are characterised by short stature and spinal abnormalities. The changes are principally in the vertebral bodies and the epiphyses of the long bones, particularly at the upper end of the femur, but mild metaphyseal involvement occurs in some types. Two forms of S.E.D. are generally recognised, the 'congenita' type in which abnormalities are present at birth, and the 'tarda' type in which the features become manifest in later childhood. Atypical forms of S.E.D. are relatively common and it is likely that the disorder is very heterogeneous.

6.1.1 Spondyloepiphyseal Dysplasia Congenita

Clinical Features

There is short trunk dwarfism with a barrel chest and marked lumbar lordosis, and genu valgum or varum may occur. The hands and feet are normal in contradistinction to the Morquio syndrome (MPS IV) to which S.E.D. has a marked clinical resemblance. Clubfoot and cleft palate may be present and many patients have eye problems in the form of myopia or retinal detachment. In the adult the weight-bearing joints, especially the hips, frequently show premature degenerative changes.

Radiographic Appearances

In the newborn there is a lack of ossification of the pubic bones and the epiphyses around the knee joint are not visible. The vertebral bodies are flat and have a pear-shaped appearance on the lateral projection. In childhood delay in the development of ossification centres continues; this is particularly marked at the hip and results in dysplasia of the femoral head and neck, with marked coxa vara. Flattening and delayed ossification of the vertebrae persist and the odontoid process is hypoplastic. In the adult the vertebral bodies are irregular and flat, the spine is short and kyphoscoliosis often develops. Shortening of the tubular bones is variable but is usually of a minor degree. The epiphyses of the proximal long bones are most severely involved, while the extremities are virtually normal.

Genetics

The classic form of S.E.D. congenita is transmitted as an autosomal dominant.

Management

Current views on the management of S.E.D. congenita have been summarised by Bailey (1973) and Kopits (1976). Odontoid hypoplasia can lead to atlanto-axial instability which may jeopardise the spinal cord. Loss of endurance, failure to walk satisfactorily when adequate neuromuscular development is present, and unexplained episodes of temporary respiratory arrest may be the earliest signs of cervical myelopathy. Occipito-cervical fusion should be carried out if there are established physical signs indicating cord compression or if CT (computerised tomography) scanning demonstrates potential compromise of the cord.

The varus deformity of the hips is responsible for the waddling gait and valgus osteotomy has been carried out to improve this problem. Arthrography is useful in the assessment of the state of the femoral heads, which ossify late.

Osteotomy about the knee may be required in the presence of valgus or varus deformity to correctly align weight-bearing through the joint and to improve walking.

6.1.2 Spondyloepiphyseal Dysplasia Tarda

Clinical Features

Appearances are variable and the most mildly affected may have no obvious clinical changes. However, by mid-childhood relative shortness of the trunk is usually present. The limbs are relatively normal but mild sternal protrusion may be seen. Back pain in childhood is sometimes the presenting feature, while in the adult premature degenerative changes may occur in the major joints, particularly in the hip.

Radiographic Appearances

There is generalised platyspondyly, with a pathognomonic 'humped' appearance of the postero-superior portion of the vertebral bodies when seen on the lateral view. The femoral necks tend to be short and mild dysplastic changes are present in the proximal large joints.

Genetics

S.E.D. tarda is inherited as an X-linked recessive.

Management

Back pain and stiffness should be treated by the standard conservative measures of a firm bed, exercises, or a spinal support. Degenerative changes in the hips may develop in early adulthood and replacement arthroplasty may be required.

6.2 Pseudoachondroplasia

Pseudoachondroplasia was initially grouped with S.E.D. and at one time was termed 'pseudoachondroplastic spondyloepiphyseal dysplasia'. This cumbersome designation has now been shortened to 'pseudoachondroplasia'. There are several forms of the disorder with considerable variation in severity, but they share the common features of involvement of the spine and the growth of the tubular bones.

Clinical Features (Fig. 6.1)

A variable degree of short-limbed dwarfism is the principal feature and patients have a superficial resemblance to achondroplasts, but the normal craniofacial appearance permits distinction. Spinal changes are variable but some degree of malalignment is usually present. Genu valgum or varum may occur and joint hypermobility, which particularly affects the wrists and fingers, is commonly encountered. The diagnosis is usually established after delayed walking and growth retardation draw attention to the underlying skeletal dysplasia.

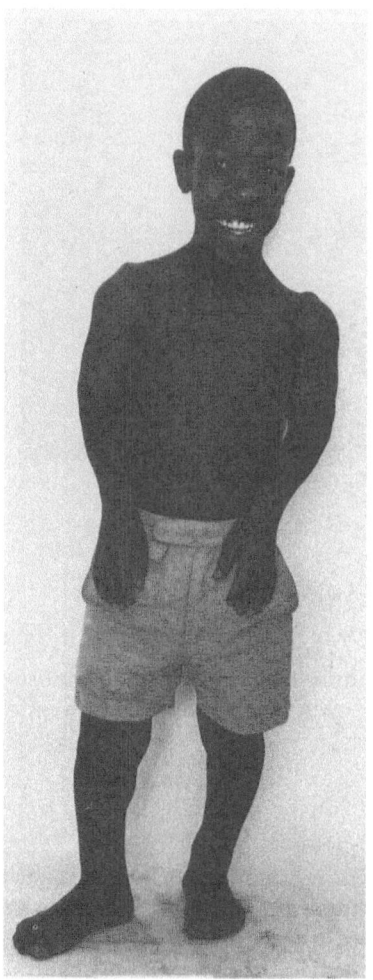

Fig. 6.1. Pseudoachondroplasia. Normal cranio-facial appearance with short-limbed dwarfism.

Radiographic Appearances (Fig. 6.2)

The radiographic abnormalities are first seen in late infancy and evolve throughout childhood. The vertebral bodies are flattened and biconvex, with irregularity of the end-plates. By adolescence the vertebral outlines appear more normal but the spinal changes vary greatly in different forms of the condition. The pelvis shows hypoplasia of the pubis and ischium, with flattening and irregularity of the acetabulae. The epiphyses of the long bones are irregular and their metaphyses are splayed and cup-shaped. The tubular bones are short and relatively broad.

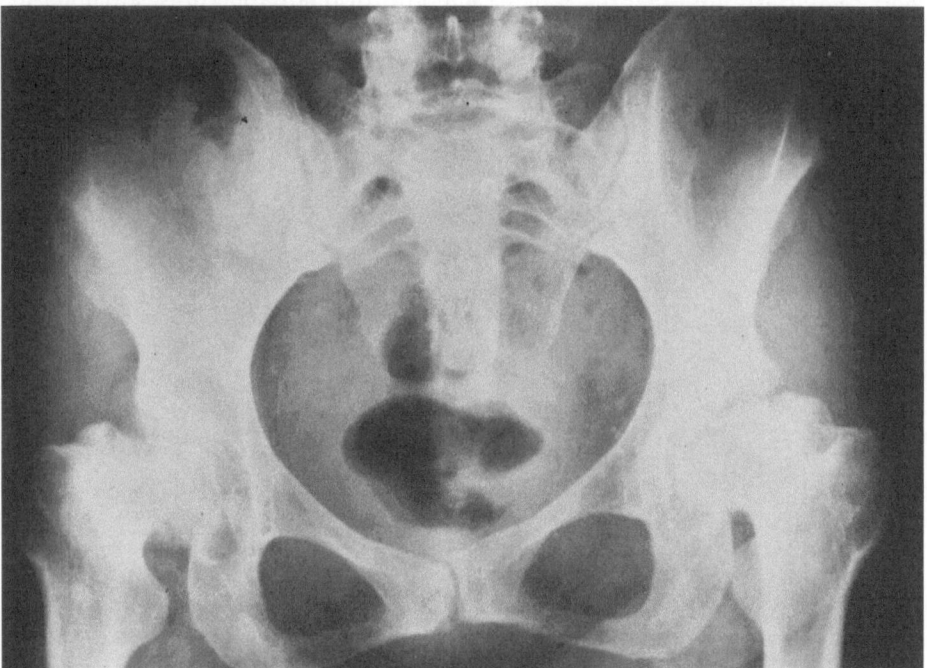

Fig. 6.2. Pseudoachondroplasia. Flattening and irregularity of the femoral heads with short varus necks.

Genetics

Pseudoachondroplasia is heterogeneous and both autosomal dominant and autosomal recessive forms have been described. These have each been subdivided into mild and severe types but delineation is incomplete.

Management

Kopits (1976), reviewing the management of 31 patients with pseudoachondroplasia, noted that deformities of the hip and knee were common in childhood and that the 'windswept' deformity of a valgus knee and adducted hip on one side and a varus knee and abducted hip on the other was often present. He advised tibial or femoral

osteotomies to ensure correct vertical alignment and thus prevent secondary dislocation of the hip, scoliosis, or permanent deformity at the knees. He emphasised the
importance of arthrograms in the evaluation of the state of unossified epiphyses.
Ligamentous laxity made assessment of the correct angle for osteotomy at operation
difficult, and repeated procedures were often required. Provided correct lower limb
alignment was maintained scoliosis was not usually severe or difficult to manage.

Although odontoid hypoplasia is frequently found in pseudoachondroplasia and
careful assessment of the degree of atlanto-axial instability is required, Kopits had
needed to perform only one occipitocervical fusion in his series.

Late degenerative changes may occur in both hips and knees and replacement
arthroplasty may be indicated (Fig. 6.3).

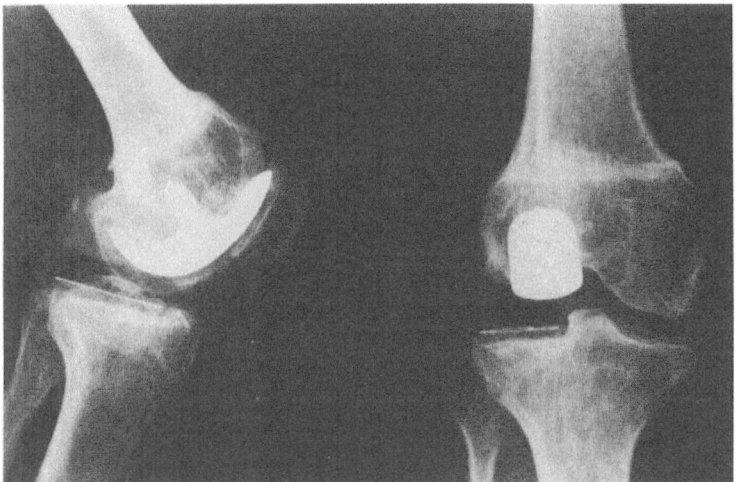

Fig. 6.3. Hemiarthroplasty of the knee in pseudoachondroplasia.

6.3 Diastrophic Dysplasia

Diastrophic dysplasia is associated with profound dwarfism and severe disability and
is one of the few inherited skeletal disorders in which the diagnosis can be made on
clinical grounds alone.

Clinical Features (Fig. 6.4)

The term 'diastrophic' is derived from the Greek word meaning twisted, tortuous or
crooked, and describes the deformities of the limbs, extremities, and spine. The
diagnosis can be made at birth on recognition of the short limbs, stiff equinus feet and
proximally set 'hitchhiker' thumbs. The palate is often cleft and the pinnae of the ears
show cystic swelling.

Some joints may be lax in infancy, but in later childhood joint contractures and
stiffness, particularly of the hips, knees, hands, and feet, present major problems.

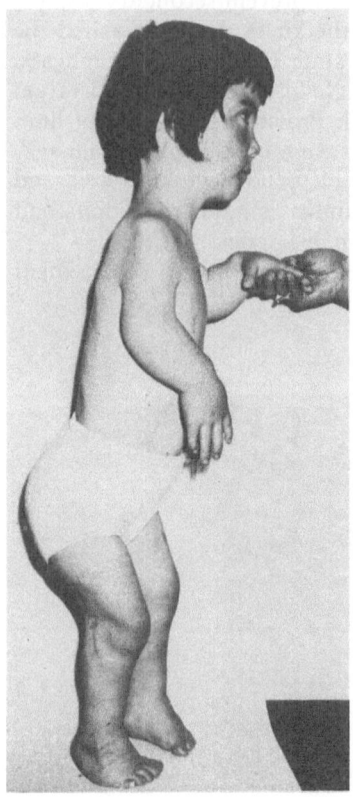

Fig. 6.4. Diastrophic dysplasia. Severe dwarfing with hitchhiker thumbs, joint contractures, rigid equinus feet, and abnormal pinnae.

Scoliosis or kyphoscoliosis is often severe and cord compression may occur. Mobility may be severely impaired by the rigid foot deformities. Individuals with diastrophic dysplasia are very dwarfed and deformed, but their intelligence is normal and there are no systemic abnormalities.

Radiographic Appearances (Figs. 6.5, 6.6)

In infancy the epiphyses of the tubular bones are flat, and the metaphyses become flared in early childhood. The hands have wide metacarpals, particularly the first, which may appear ovoid, and the phalanges are shorter and broader than normal. Carpal ossification is irregular. Similar abnormalities are seen in the foot, where the equinus deformity predominates. The hip joints show characteristic changes with wide acetabulae, flat irregular femoral heads with short wide varus necks, and prominent greater trochanters. A cone-shaped deformity in the lower femoral metaphysis allows accommodation of a deformed epiphysis. The spine may be normal at birth but progressive kyphoscoliosis often develops during infancy and may become very severe.

Genetics

Diastrophic dysplasia is inherited as an autosomal recessive trait.

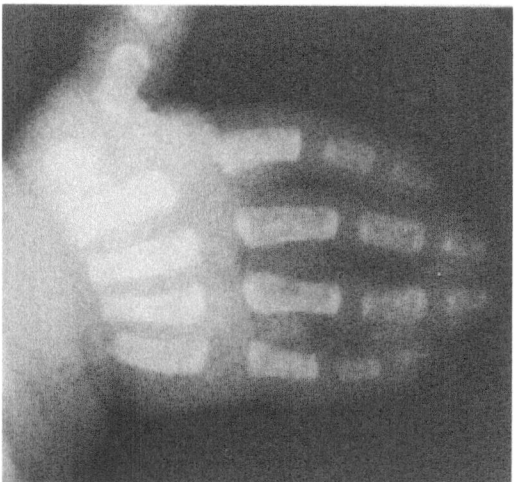

Fig. 6.5. Diastrophic dysplasia. Hand of an infant showing broad tubular bones and ovoid first metacarpal with hitchhiker thumb.

Fig. 6.6. Diastrophic dwarfism. AP view of pelvis showing wide acetabulae, flattened femoral heads, coxa vara, and prominent greater trochanters.

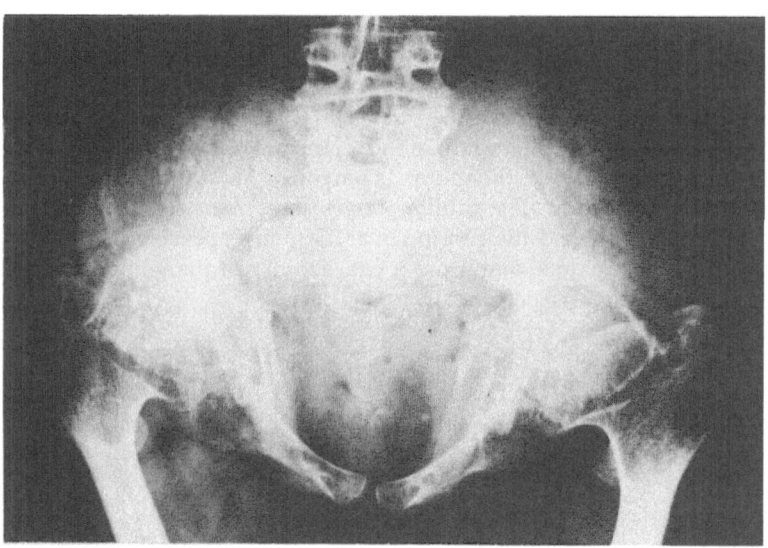

Management

The management of the skeletal problems has been fully reviewed by Bailey (1973) and Kopits (1976). The severe clubfoot deformities present the principal difficulty and early soft tissue release may give the best chance of obtaining correction, although Kopits considers that unless the flexion contractures of the hip and knee are also dealt with recurrence of equinus is inevitable. Late operations have usually proved valueless. Untreated patients manage fairly well with special shoes but reliance on crutches may be necessary for reasonable mobility.

Both scoliosis and kyphosis may be severe in diastrophic dysplasia and since in this disorder little spinal growth occurs after the age of ten, early spinal fusion is recommended. Spinal cord compression is sometimes encountered and decompression may be required for spinal stenosis.

Patients adapt well to their hand disabilities and attempts to improve function by operation are not usually warranted.

Early osteoarthritis of the hips commonly occurs and may require replacement arthroplasty.

6.4 Metatropic Dysplasia

Clinical Features

Metatropic dysplasia presents at birth with short limbs and a trunk of normal length, but in late infancy a rapidly progressive kyphoscoliosis results in short trunk dwarfism. The limbs have bulbous, stiff joints, and stubby hands and feet which are hypermobile. A tail-like skin fold, which is sometimes present overlying the sacrum, is a useful diagnostic indicator. Cardio-respiratory problems cause a significant infant mortality but survival into early adulthood is not uncommon. The effects of the severe progressive scoliosis and atlanto-axial instability are potentially fatal.

Radiographic Appearances

Characteristic radiographic changes are present at birth. There is defective ossification of the vertebral bodies which are flat or diamond shaped in the lateral projection. The intervertebral spaces appear wide, the thorax is narrowed and the ribs are short, with flared costochondral junctions. The tubular bones show marked metaphyseal expansion, resembling bar-bells, and the epiphyses are late in appearing, becoming deformed and flattened. The proximal femur has a characteristic square appearance. With increasing age kyphoscoliosis becomes very marked.

Genetics

Metatropic dysplasia is inherited as an autosomal recessive.

Management

Cervical cord compression due to atlanto-axial instability may be present from an early age, and stabilisation of the upper cervical spine is then indicated. Conservative treatment of the rapidly advancing kyphoscoliosis has proved profitless and early reduction and fusion are warranted. The hips are usually painless and stable but correction of knee contractures may be of value.

6.5 Spondylometaphyseal Dysplasia (S.M.D.)

The spondylometaphyseal dysplasias (S.M.D.) are a heterogeneous group of inherited disorders in which abnormalities in the vertebral bodies and metaphyses of the long bones predominate. Collectively the S.M.D.s are comparatively common but there is considerable variation in the clinical and radiological appearances of the different forms. Some epiphyseal involvement may be present and if this is significant the designation 'spondylo-epi-metaphyseal dysplasia' (S.E.M.D.) is used; this condition is also heterogeneous.

Clinical Features

Disproportionate short stature is present in both S.M.D. and S.E.M.D. The head, face, and intelligence are normal and changes are confined to the skeletal system. Genu valgus and varus often occur, while spinal complications range from mild malalignment to severe kyphoscoliosis, with cardio-respiratory failure and cord compression. Generalised joint laxity distinguishes one form of S.E.M.D. and may lead to multiple dislocations and progressive spinal deformity.

Radiographic Appearances

Joint dislocation, especially of the elbows, deformity of the knees, and spinal malalignment may be evident. The skull is normal apart from mild hypoplasia of the facial bones. Platyspondyly is severe and the anterior portions of the vertebrae are pointed (Fig. 6.7). The metaphyses of the tubular bones are irregular and changes of variable degree are seen in the epiphyses. In the pelvis, the iliac wings are squared, while the femoral necks are short (Fig. 6.8).

Genetics

S.M.D. and S.E.M.D. are very heterogeneous and autosomal dominant and recessive forms of each have been recorded.

Management

Deformities of the lower limb are managed by corrective osteotomy. Should spinal malalignment develop, regular surveillance is mandatory since if progression of the curves becomes rapid, fusion will be required.

In the form of S.E.M.D. which is associated with generalised joint laxity, kyphoscoliosis is usually progressive and severe and management may be very difficult. The majority of these patients require spinal fusion and repeated procedures may be necessary.

6.6 Other Disorders

6.6.1 Parastremmatic Dysplasia

Parastremmatic dysplasia is a rare disorder in which there is dwarfism with a severe fixed kyphoscoliosis and knobbly, bowed limbs with stiff contracted joints. The radiographic appearances are unmistakable; the long bones have curved diaphyses, while the metaphyses are greatly expanded and the epiphyses irregular and late in appearing. The expanded ends of the long bones have a curious flocculated appearance which is also seen in the grossly distorted pelvis and kyphoscoliotic spine. The pattern of inheritance is uncertain.

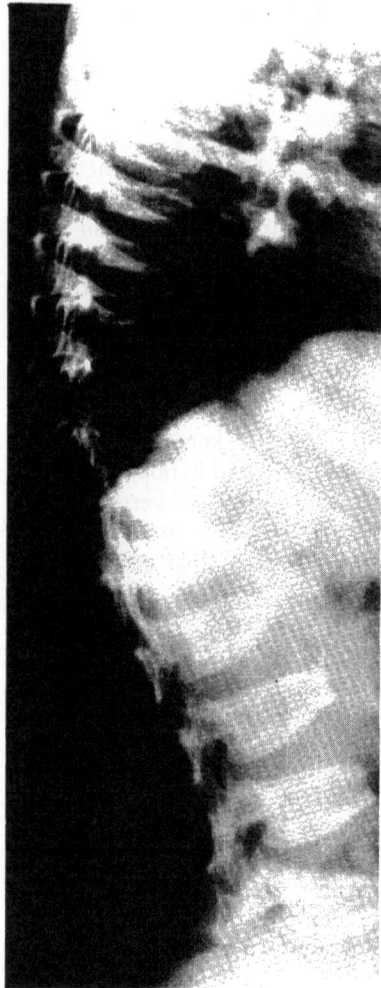

Fig. 6.7. Spondylometaphyseal dysplasia. Thoracic kyphosis and platyspondyly; the vertebral bodies are pointed anteriorly. From Koslowski et al. 1981.

6.6.2 Dyggve-Melchior-Clausen Syndrome

The Dyggve-Melchior-Clausen syndrome has many features in common with the Morquio syndrome (MPS IV) and is characterised by dwarfing, a coarse facies, and mental retardation. Details of about 20 patients have been reported, the majority of whom have been of Lebanese stock. Radiographs show marked platyspondyly with anterior projection of the middle third of the vertebral bodies and a pathognomonic irregular configuration of the iliac crest. Inheritance is autosomal recessive.

6.6.3 Kniest Dysplasia

Kniest disease is a rare disorder which resembles metatropic dysplasia. The syndrome may be apparent clinically at birth or in early infancy. The main characteristics are dwarfism with a flat mid-face, depressed nasal bridge, short broad

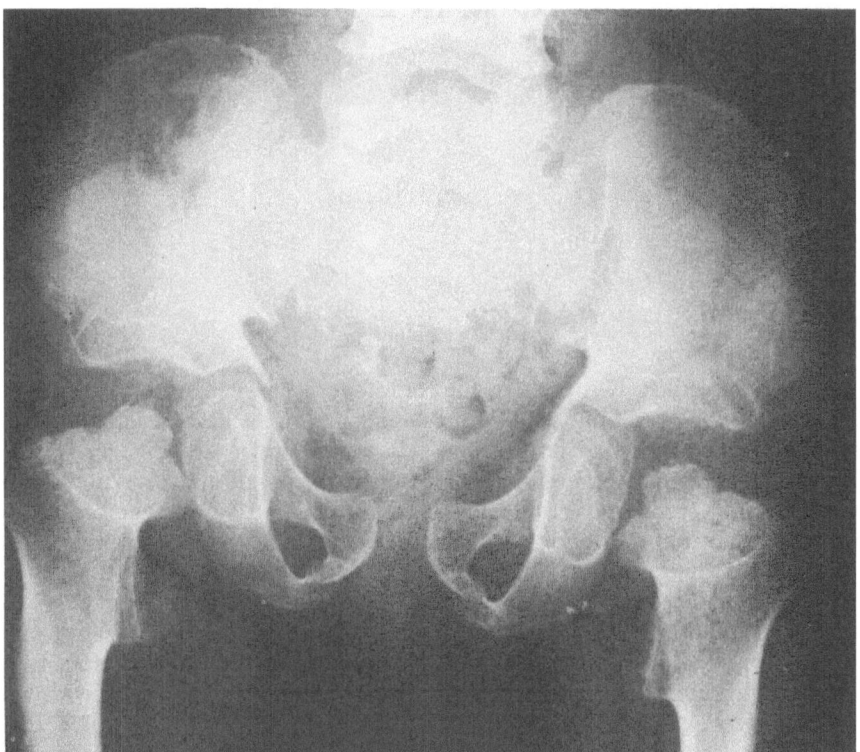

Fig. 6.8. Spondylometaphyseal dysplasia. The iliac wings are squared and the sacro-iliac notches are shortened. The acetabular roofs are narrow and the femoral necks wide and short. From Koslowski et al. 1981.

thorax, short curved limbs and a crouching gait. There is an exaggerated lumbar lordosis with flexion contractures of the hips. Cleft palate, deafness and myopia are frequent concomitants. A mild kyphoscoliosis is usually present but may become progressive. Stabilisation of the upper cervical spine is sometimes necessary as odontoid hypoplasia predisposes to atlanto-axial instability. The radiographs show marked platyspondyly with irregular vertebral bodies. The pelvis is broad with a narrow inlet and the acetabulae are enlarged and grossly irregular with a honey-combed appearance. The femoral capital epiphyses appear very late and the heads may remain unossified throughout childhood. The trochanteric region is greatly expanded and flattened and the femoral neck is short. The tubular bones are short and dumb-bell shaped with enlarged metaphyses. Inheritance is autosomal dominant.

References

Spondyloepiphyseal Dysplasia Congenita, Pseudoachondroplasia and Diastrophic Dysplasia

Bailey JA II (1973) Disproportionate short stature. Saunders, Philadelphia London Toronto
Kopits SE (1976) Orthopaedic complications of dwarfism. Clin Orthop 114:153

7. Generalised Decrease in Bone Density

7.1 Osteogenesis Imperfecta

Osteogenesis imperfecta (OI) is perhaps the commonest inherited skeletal dysplasia. Since the basic defect is an abnormality of the collagen other tissues, including the teeth, skin, tendons, ligaments, fasciae and sclerae, may also be affected.

Osteogenesis imperfecta has been known for many years and the large number of cases available for study have resulted in comprehensive investigation of the syndrome. It is clear that the condition is heterogeneous, and that the severity of the stigmata is very variable in the different forms.

The disorder has been broadly categorised on a clinical basis into a severe 'congenita' form, which is evident at birth, and a milder 'tarda' type in which problems arise in childhood. Three types are distinguishable by radiographic study ('thick' bone, 'thin' bone and 'cystic' bone), but these appearances change with age and their diagnostic value is uncertain.

There have been considerable problems in classifying OI, but following a comprehensive survey in Victoria, Australia, Sillence et al. (1979) suggested that there were at least four distinct forms, as shown below:

Type	Clinical features	Mode of inheritance
1	Blue sclerae. Moderate tendency to fracture	Autosomal dominant (heterogeneous)
2	Perinatal lethality	Autosomal recessive
3	White sclerae. Dwarfism, severe bone fragility and deformity	Autosomal recessive
4	White sclerae. Moderate tendency to fracture	Autosomal dominant

Notwithstanding this heterogeneity, retention of the congenita and tarda grouping is useful for descriptive purposes, although these are artificial categories which do not bear any close relationship to the specific fundamental defect.

7.1.1 Osteogenesis Imperfecta Congenita

Clinical Features

At birth disproportionate shortening of the limbs is obvious, and the head is large with a soft calvarium and wide fontanelles. Many babies with this type of OI are stillborn or only survive for a few days with death usually occurring from intra-cranial haemorrhage. Survivors who reach adulthood are often dwarfed with severe skeletal deformity.

Radiographic Appearances

There is poor ossification of the calvarium with wide sutures and numerous wormian bones. Multiple fractures of the ribs and long bones may be seen. The vertebrae are normal at birth but if the infant survives they become soft and flattened or biconcave, and spinal deformities arise. The limb bones vary in appearance. In the 'thick bone' type the bones are short and wide, but in the 'thin bone' type the shafts are slender with thin cortices and marked osteoporosis. The epiphyses are normal and the metaphyses may be expanded.

Genetics

The majority of neonates with OI congenita have normal parents and may represent new mutations for a dominant gene. A proportion, however, have an autosomal recessive condition and the presence of multiple rib fractures and thick 'concertina' tubular bones may be diagnostic of this form.

7.1.2 Osteogenesis Imperfecta Tarda

Clinical Features (Fig. 7.1)

In OI tarda problems with bone fragility do not arise before early childhood. Thereafter fractures may occur regularly, with some patients having many but others few until the tendency diminishes in adulthood. Fracture healing is rapid and usually uncomplicated, but the occasional patient develops hyperplastic callus and doubts sometimes arise concerning the possibility of osteomyelitis or osteosarcoma.

The face is triangular and there is an increase in the bitemporal diameter. The sclerae are characteristically blue, but the shade varies with age and ethnic pigmentation, and in at least two uncommon, severe varieties of OI, the sclerae are white. A bruising tendency, abnormalities of the teeth and ligamentous laxity may be present. Otosclerosis and deafness develop in adulthood in about 20% of patients. Loss of height occurs due to vertebral collapse and some degree of scoliosis may be present (Benson 1978).

Radiographic Appearances (Figs. 7.2–7.5)

Generalised demineralisation of the skeleton is seen and the long bones are gracile and deformed, due to softening and bending of their shafts or to malunion following fracture. Ossification of the cranial vault is retarded, with a bitemporal bulge and wormian bones in the sutures. The vertebral bodies show platyspondyly and are biconcave.

Genetics

The majority of patients with OI tarda have a condition which is inherited as an autosomal dominant. There is considerable heterogeneity but clear-cut biochemical categorisation of the various types has not yet been established. The sclerae are white in the uncommon severe autosomal dominant and autosomal recessive forms, but are blue in the more usual autosomal dominant form which is relatively benign.

Management (Fig. 7.6)

A major object of management is to minimise deformity during childhood since the tendency to fracture greatly decreases after adolescence. Fractures which are treated conservatively require careful splinting with meticulous attention to detail. Early mobilisation is important to lessen osteoporosis induced by rest.

In view of the fragility of the bone, movement must be made as safe as possible in childhood, when fracture is most likely. The limbs and spine may be protected by splints, which must fit accurately, be comfortable and easily moved. A vacuum casting technique is useful in making splints of this type (Nichols and Strange 1972) and quick-setting polymers, such as Neoprakt, are useful orthotic materials. Aids such as an electric wheelchair and tailored slings for lifting are required for ease of movement.

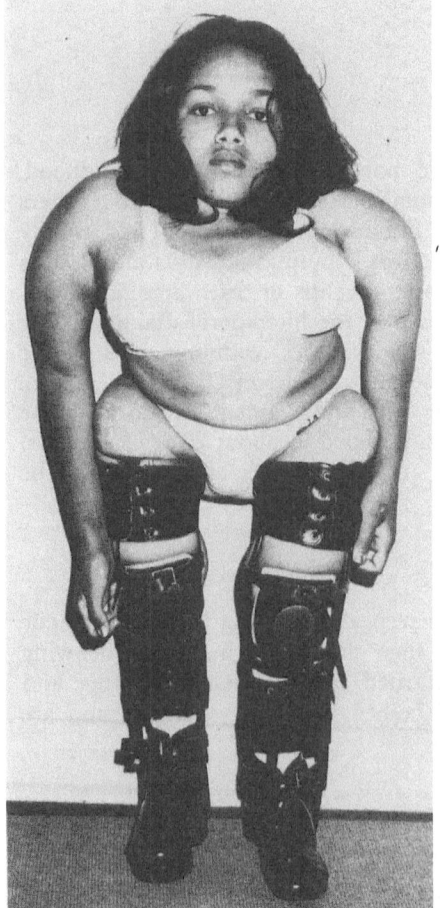

Fig. 7.1. Osteogenesis imperfecta. Severe dwarfing in a young woman with an autosomal recessive form. She has a gross kyphoscoliosis and braces support her lower limbs which had suffered many fractures.

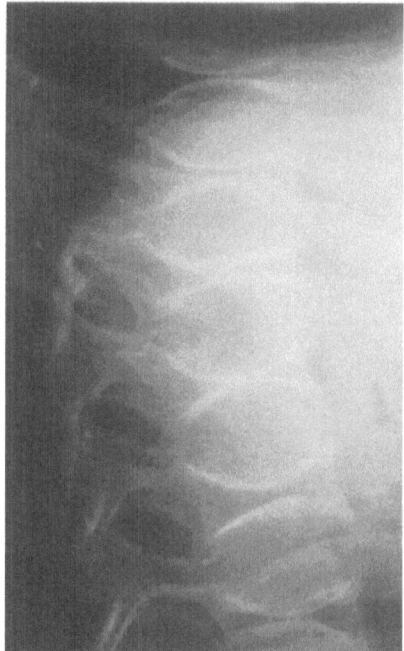

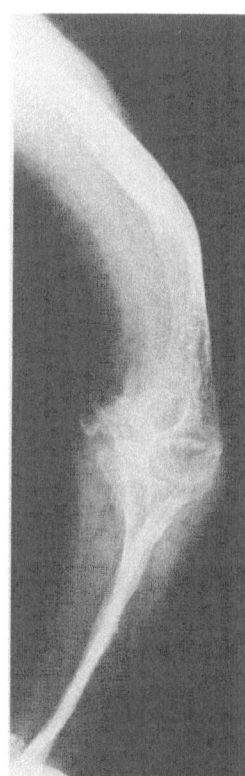

Fig. 7.2. Osteogenesis imperfecta.
Platyspondyly with biconcave vertebrae.

Fig. 7.3. Osteogenesis imperfecta. The humerus is bowed and undermineralised. The cortex is thin and sites of healed fractures are apparent. The forearm bones are gracile and hypoplastic.

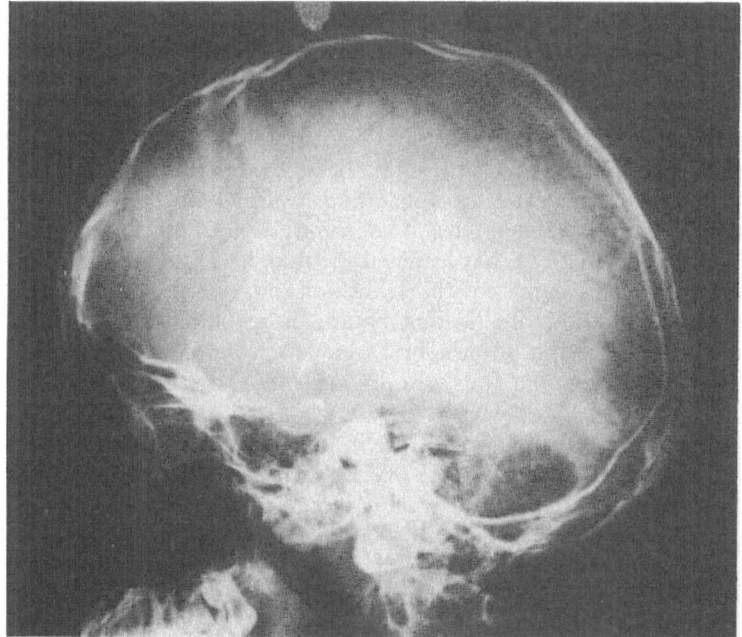

Fig. 7.4. Lateral view of skull in OI tarda (courtesy of Professor S. P. F. Hughes, Edinburgh).

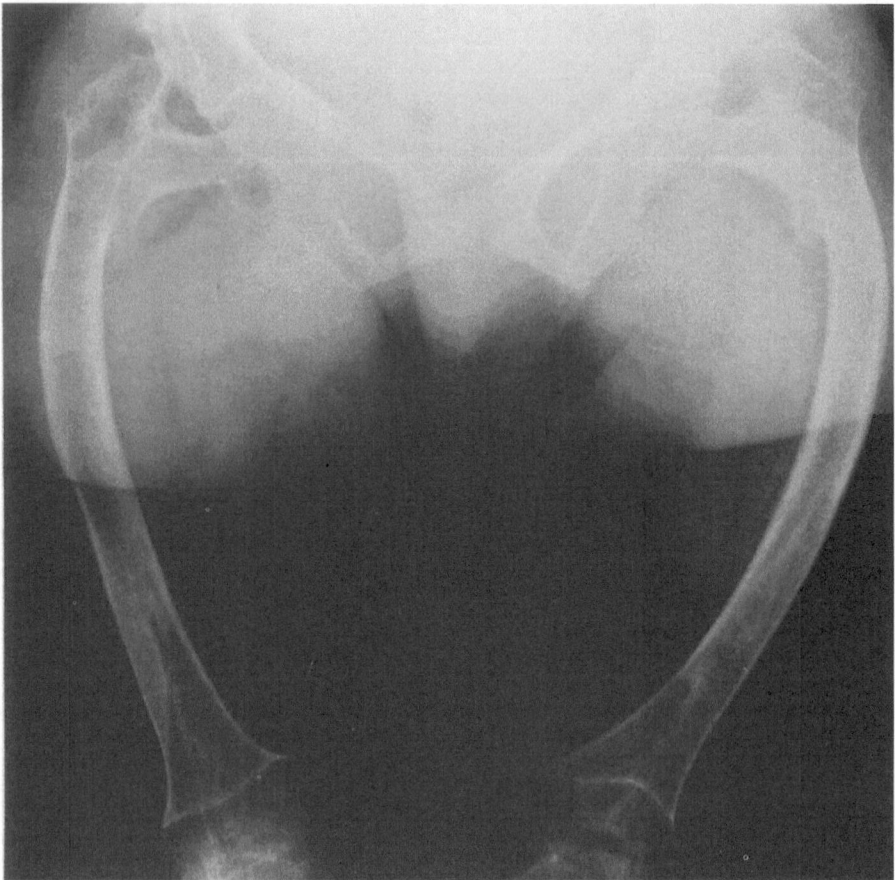

Fig. 7.5. Osteogenesis imperfecta. Femoral bowing but no evidence of fracture.

The fragmentation, realignment, and intramedullary fixation of long bones, especially of the lower limb, as advocated by Sofeld and Miller (1959) have greatly improved the management of the fragile bones. The introduction of the sliding rod, pioneered by Bailey and Dubow (1965), has lessened the number of revision nailing procedures which are required during growth. Marafioti and Westin (1977) published a review of 153 rod fixations in 72 long bones, using both standard and expanding rods. They commented that the Bailey-Dubow rod 'represents a measurably improvement over non-elongating rods'. Rodriguez (1976) reached a similar conclusion.

The incidence of some degree of spinal curvature in patients over 12 years of age approaches 80% according to Benson et al. (1978). In their series the curves were mild in all children below 8 years of age, and curves of more than 8° were seen only in children over the age of 12 years. When a curve was noted in early life progression was to be expected. The curves were worse in patients with OI congenita and in those who were confined to a wheelchair. These authors found that the Milwaukee brace usually failed to control the curve and they advised early spinal fusion with or without Harrington rod instrumentation. Renshaw et al. (1979) reviewed 54 patients and agreed that the scoliosis was worse in children with the severe forms of OI. They

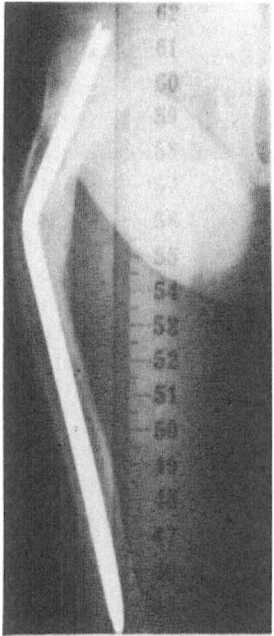
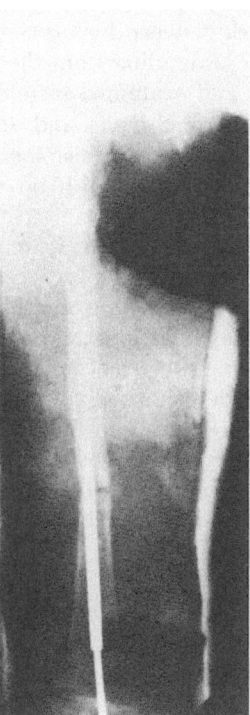
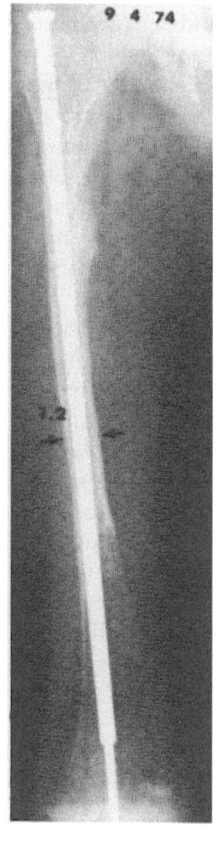
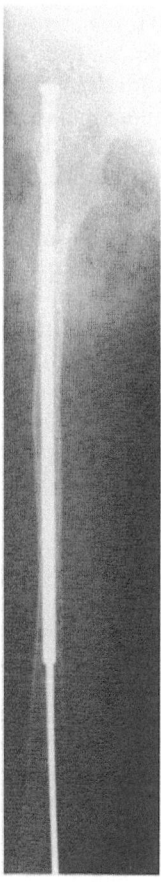

Pre-operative appearance
with bent intramedullary
nail.

Immediately after insertion
of Bailey Dubow telescoping
rod.

2 years after
operation.

4 years after
operation.

Fig. 7.6. The Bailey Dubow telescoping rod in Osteogenesis imperfecta. (Reproduced by courtesy of R. B. Gledhill MD, Montreal Children's Hospital, Montreal PQ, Canada)

concluded that progression of the deformity was likely and that its rate of deterioration paralleled the normal growth curve. Attempts at arrest of progression of the scoliosis by bracing were usually fruitless and they advised early fusion. Similar views were expressed by Moe et al. (1978). In reviewing their results of operation for scoliosis in eight patients Cristofaro et al. (1979) emphasised that because of the poor quality of the bone spinal instrumentation could not be used to obtain correction of the curve but only for stabilisation. They used a plastic body jacket for post-operative care and had obtained fusion in between 9 and 12 months. They reported no loss of correction in their patients when reviewed 1 year after operation.

The presence of hyperplastic callus may pose a diagnostic problem because its clinical features may be similar to those of osteosarcoma or osteomyelitis. However, the incidence of hyperplastic callus formation appears to be low since Benson et al. (1978) recorded only three instances in their study of 143 patients. Similarly, the frequency of osteosarcoma in OI is probably no greater than in the general population, and Rutkowski et al. (1979) could find only nine cases recorded in the world literature. Routine laboratory tests, radiographs, tomographs, bone scans, and CT scans are insufficient to distinguish between hyperplastic callus and osteosarcoma, and an adequate section of tissue, extending from the overlying muscles to the underlying bone, should be removed and examined histologically if this diagnostic dilemma arises. Hyperplastic callus is gelatinous and semi-cartilaginous with a macroscopic resemblance to chondrosarcoma, but histological examination shows a fibro-mucoid cartilage-like tissue or chondroid, with no evidence of a malignant stroma.

Many medical regimens have been tried in OI, including drugs, diet and radiotherapy, but none have been successful. There is currently no therapeutic agent which can be recommended for clinical use, but recent evidence suggests that long-term treatment with calcitonin may be helpful. Rosenberg et al. (1977) treated four patients with OI congenita with long courses of calcitonin and showed that their bone mass did not decrease with respect to normal controls, as occurred in patients who did not receive calcitonin. There was no difference between treated and untreated patients with OI tarda. Attempts have been made to assess the effectiveness of calcitonin in patients with OI by comparing the number of fractures sustained in treated patients with those who were not treated, but the many variable factors associated with injury make it difficult to gauge the influence of a drug and no clear-cut results have emerged.

Few fractures occur after the age of 16, and most patients adapt well to their condition and become productive members of society (Moorefield and Miller 1980).

7.2 Idiopathic Osteolysis

Reports of patients with 'disappearing bones' have been published since the middle of the 19th century. Osteolysis can occur in the presence of infection or rheumatoid disease, in association with disorders of the central nervous system such as tabes, syringomyelia and leprosy, and as a result of massive local haemangiomata. There is an idiopathic group of osteolysis in which no causative factor can be detected.

Idiopathic osteolysis can be classified into three broad categories:

1) In the first type onset is usually in childhood, and the phalanges are always affected. Painful swelling of the digits is the earliest physical manifestation and bony collapse and deformity follow, with more widespread skeletal changes in some patients. Autosomal dominant and autosomal recessive inheritance has been recorded in addition to non-genetic forms of the disorder.

2) In the second group the tarso-carpal regions are prominently involved. This was the principal site of involvement in three generations of one family (Gluck and Miller 1972), while in other kindreds the bony distribution has been more widespread. Tarso-carpal osteolysis in association with nephropathy has also been reported (Shurtleef et al. 1964; Torg and Steel 1968).

3) This group is characterised by the destruction of all or part of a bone by angiomatous tissue and has been known by various eponyms such as 'massive osteolysis', 'vanishing' or 'phantom' bone disease and Gorham's disease. The process may spread insidiously, involving adjacent bones and soft tissues, or spontaneous arrest may occur (Sage and Allen 1974; Campbell et al. 1975). This form of idiopathic osteolysis is neither inherited nor congenital.

Management

There is no general agreement as to the management of this disorder. Surgical treatment of long bone osteolysis has consisted of amputation or local resection, with or without replacement prostheses or bone grafts (Sage and Allen 1974; Burrows et al. 1975). The use of radiotherapy has been advocated (Johnson and McClure 1958) but the results appear to be equivocal.

References

Osteogenesis Imperfecta

Bailey RW, Dubow HI (1965) Experimental and clinical studies of longitudinal bone growth—utilizing a new method of internal fixation across the epiphyseal plate. J Bone Joint Surg [Am] 47:1669 Proceedings of the American Orthopaedic Association.

Benson DR, Donaldson DH, Millar EA (1978) The spine in osteogenesis imperfecta. J Bone Joint Surg [Am] 60:925

Cristofaro RL, Hoek KJ, Bonnett CA, Brown JC (1979) Operative treatment of spinal deformity in O.I. Clin Orthop 139:40

Marafioti RL, Westin GW (1977) Elongating intramedullary rods in the treatment of osteogenesis imperfecta. J Bone Joint Surg [Am] 59:467

Moe JH, Winter RB, Bradford DS, Lonstein JE (1978) Scoliosis and other spinal deformities. Saunders, Philadelphia, p 607

Moorefield WG Jnr., Miller GR (1980) Aftermath of osteogenesis imperfecta: the disease in adulthood. J Bone Joint Surg [Am] 62:113

Nichols PJR, Strange TV (1972) A method of casting severely deformed and disabled patients. Rheumatology and Physical Medicine 11:356

Renshaw TS, Cook RS, Albright JA (1979) Scoliosis in osteogenesis imperfecta. Clin Orthop 145:163

Rodriguez RP (1976) Report of multiple osteotomies and intramedullary fixation by an extensible intramedullary device in children with osteogenesis imperfecta. Clin Orthop 116:261

Rosenberg E, Lang R, Boisseau V, Rojanasathit S, Avioli LV (1977) Effect of long term calcitonin therapy on the clinical course of osteogenesis imperfecta. J Clin Endocrinol Metab 44:346

Rutkowski R, Resnick P, McMaster JH (1979) Osteosarcoma occurring in osteogenesis imperfecta. J Bone Joint Surg [Am] 61:606

Sillence DO, Senn A, Danks DM (1979) Genetic heterogeneity in osteogenesis imperfecta. J Med Genet 16:101

Sofeld HA, Millar EA (1959) Fragmentation, realignment and intramedullary rod fixation of deformities of the long bones in children. A ten-year appraisal. J Bone Joint Surg [Am] 41:1371

Idiopathic Osteolysis

Burrows HJ, Wilson JN, Scales JT (1975) Excision of tumours of the humerus and femur, with restoration by internal prostheses. J Bone Joint Surg [Br] 57:148

Campbell J, Almond HGA, Johnson R (1975) Massive osteolysis of the humerus with spontaneous recovery. J Bone Joint Surg [Br] 57:238

Gluck J, Miller JJ (1972) Familial osteolysis of the carpal and tarsal bones. J Pediatr 81:506

Johnson PM, McClure JG (1958) Observations on massive osteolysis Radiology 71:28

Sage MR, Allen PW (1974) Massive osteolysis. Report of a case. J Bone Joint Surg [Br] 56:130

Shurtleff DB, Sprakes RS, Clawson K, Guntheroth WG, Mottet NK (1964) Hereditary osteolysis with hypertension and nephropathy. JAMA 188:363

Torg JS, Steel HH (1968) Essential osteolysis with nephropathy: A review of the literature and case report of an unusual syndrome. J Bone Joint Surg Br 50:1629

8. Increased Bone Density

8.1 Osteopetrosis

The terms 'osteopetrosis' or 'Albers-Schönberg disease' have been used loosely for a large number of conditions in which generalised increased radiological density of the skeleton is present. These designations are more accurately reserved for the specific dominant and recessive conditions which form the subject of this section.

Osteopetrosis is conventionally subdivided into the adult, tarda or benign autosomal dominant form, and the infantile, precocious, malignant autosomal recessive type. However, intermediate forms are not uncommon and it is sometimes difficult to assign a patient to a specific category.

8.1.1 Autosomal Recessive Form

The autosomal recessive type of osteopetrosis is very rare. In this condition stillbirth is not unusual, while the survivors fail to thrive and show spontaneous bruising, abnormal bleeding, anaemia and hepatosplenomegaly. Cranial nerve palsies, particularly of the optic, oculomotor, and facial nerves are common. Dentition is delayed and the teeth are of poor quality. Death from overwhelming infection or haemorrhage usually occurs by early childhood. The radiographic changes resemble those of the dominant form of osteopetrosis (see below). Endobones are prominent and the metaphyses of the long bones are expanded and contain transverse bands of lucency and sclerosis.

8.1.2 Autosomal Dominant Form

The autosomal dominant benign type of osteopetrosis is comparatively common and has a wide ethnic and geographical distribution.

Clinical Features

Persons with benign osteopetrosis are often free of symptoms and the diagnosis may be made by chance, following radiographic examination for other reasons. The general health is unimpaired but facial palsy and deafness may result from nerve compression by overgrowth of bone in the cranial foramina. Pathological fractures are troublesome in some patients but many do not experience this problem. Tooth extraction may be difficult and osteomyelitis of the jaw can follow this procedure. Anaemia has been reported in a few patients, but this is not a consistent complication. The variability in clinical characteristics may well be a reflection of underlying heterogeneity.

Radiographic Appearances (Figs. 8.1–8.4)

There is marked thickening and widening of the calvarium with sclerosis of the base of the skull and mandible. In the spine sclerosis is most marked in the vertebral end-plates producing the appearance of 'sandwich vertebrae' or a 'rugger jersey' spine. The cortices of the long bones are widened and sclerotic, but the bone contours are little disturbed. Involvement of the bones of the hand is variable and they are sometimes spared. In young patients the long bones may show a 'bone within a bone' or 'endobone' appearance due to central diaphyseal sclerosis.

Genetics

There is little doubt that the common adult or tarda autosomal dominant form of osteopetrosis is heterogeneous and it is likely that a rare but severe adult 'intermediate' variety is inherited as an autosomal recessive trait. The classical infantile or lethal form of osteopetrosis is an autosomal recessive.

Management

The infantile, autosomal recessive form of osteopetrosis is one of the few bone dysplasias in which there has been some progress in the search for medical treatment. Parathyroid hormone, vitamin A and vitamin D have been used in attempts to promote calcium loss, while the administration of corticosteroids and dietary restriction of calcium have aimed to decrease absorption. All such attempts have

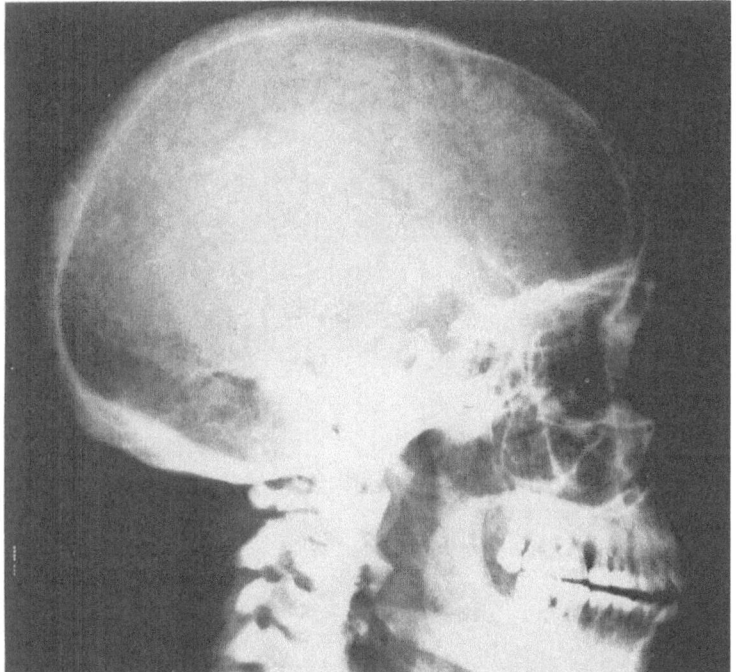

Fig. 8.1. Osteopetrosis: benign form. Lateral view of skull showing thickening of the calvarium and basal sclerosis.

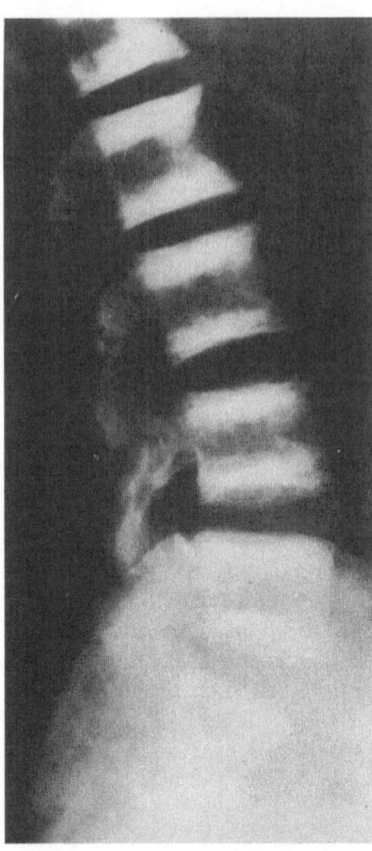

Fig. 8.2. Osteopetrosis: benign form. Lateral view of lumbar spine showing end-plate sclerosis, the rugger-jersey spine.

Fig. 8.3. Osteopetrosis: benign form. AP view of pelvis showing generalised sclerosis and cortical thickening of upper femora but with little disturbance of the overall configuration.

▼

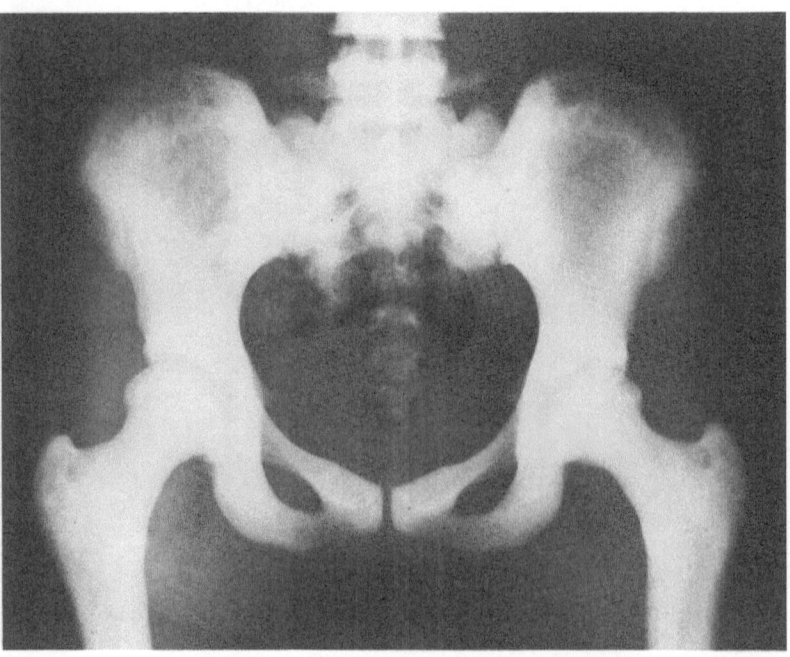

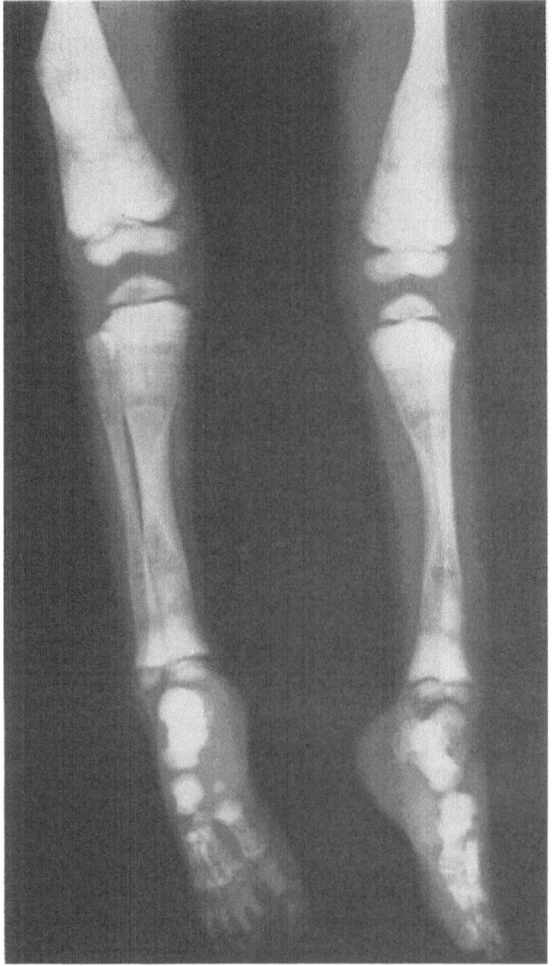

Fig. 8.4. Osteopetrosis: benign form in a young child. Metaphyseal undermodelling is apparent with transverse and vertical sclerotic bands and 'endobone' formation.

proved unsuccessful (Milhaud and Labat 1978). Shapiro et al. (1980) have recently postulated that the basic defect lies in the osteoclasts which do not respond to parathyroid hormone in the usual way. However the availability of animal models for study has improved the prospects of finding effective treatment. Walker (1973) observed that in mice osteopetrosis underwent complete remission within 6 weeks after marrow transplantation from normal siblings. Similar results were obtained in rats, and subsequently Ballet et al. (1977) gave a compatible bone marrow transfusion to a 3-month-old infant with osteopetrosis congenita. The dramatic improvement which occurred was still sustained 18 months later. Milhaud and Labat (1978) found that humoral factors produced by the thymus are involved in the remodelling of the skeleton, and suggested that osteopetrosis should be considered as an immune disorder and not merely a primary disturbance of calcium and bone metabolism.

Reeves et al. (1979) have given prednisone to infants with severe osteopetrosis to improve bone marrow function. They found that regular prednisone dosage resulted in a decrease in the size of the liver and spleen, an increase in the quantity and quality of haemopoietic tissue in the bone marrow and improvement of the anaemia.

The autosomal dominant form of osteopetrosis may present few clinical problems. However, pathological fractures may occur and treatment by traction, immobilisation in plaster casts or internal fixation is usually successful (Fig. 8.5). Reports of the state of the bone at operation for internal fixation vary between 'like chalk' and 'like marble', but extreme hardness is commonly found (Breck et al. 1975). The early onset of osteoarthritis of the hip in osteopetrosis has been reported and total hip replacement may be carried out without undue trouble, although Cameron and Dewar (1977) experienced difficulty in both acetabular and femoral reaming. The extreme hardness of the jaws makes removal of carious teeth difficult and osteomyelitis of the mandible following dental abscess is a well documented complication; hyperbaric oxygen has been successfully utilised in its treatment (Mainous et al. 1975).

Facial palsy and deafness due to cranial nerve compression may warrant operative intervention (Hamersma 1970, 1974).

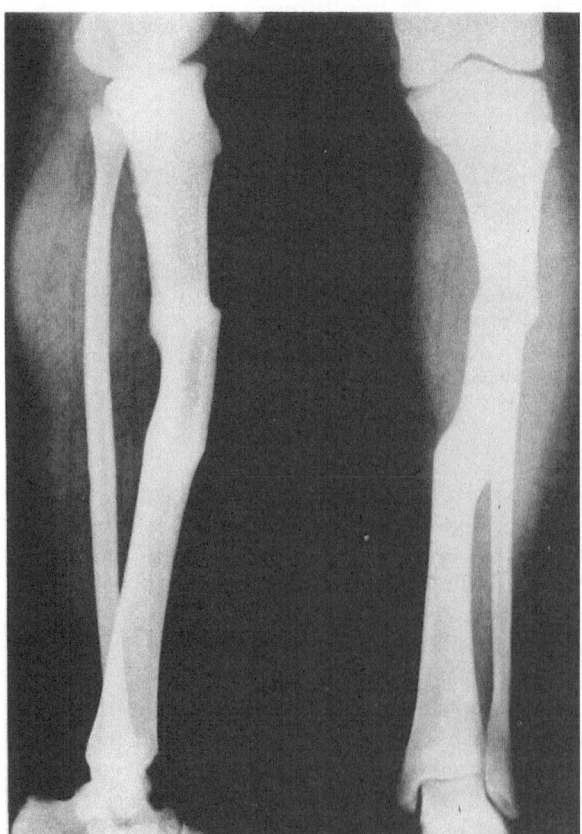

Fig. 8.5. Osteopetrosis: benign form. Healed pathological fractures in tibia of an adult.

8.2 Pycnodysostosis

This syndrome was delineated from the other sclerotic bone dysplasias in 1962 by Maroteaux and Lamy, who later postulated that the impressionist painter Toulouse Lautrec might have been affected (Maroteaux and Lamy 1965).

Clinical Features

The predominant characteristic is shortness of stature. The face is small and triangular and the mandible is underdeveloped. The hands are short and square and the terminal phalanges are stubby. Pathological fractures occur but healing is usually satisfactory. The teeth are irregular and may show early caries.

Radiographic Appearances (Figs. 8.6, 8.7 and 8.8)

There is generalised skeletal density, which may be minor in infancy but progresses thereafter. Bony modelling is not significantly abnormal. The skull shows a large calvarium with widened suture lines, persistent fontanelles and wormian bones. The facial skeleton is hypoplastic and the mandibular angle is obtuse. The terminal phalanges are short and irregular and resemble acro-osteolysis. The clavicles may show hypoplasia of their outer ends and the Madelung deformity may be present in the forearms. The long bones have sclerotic cortices with narrow medullary cavities.

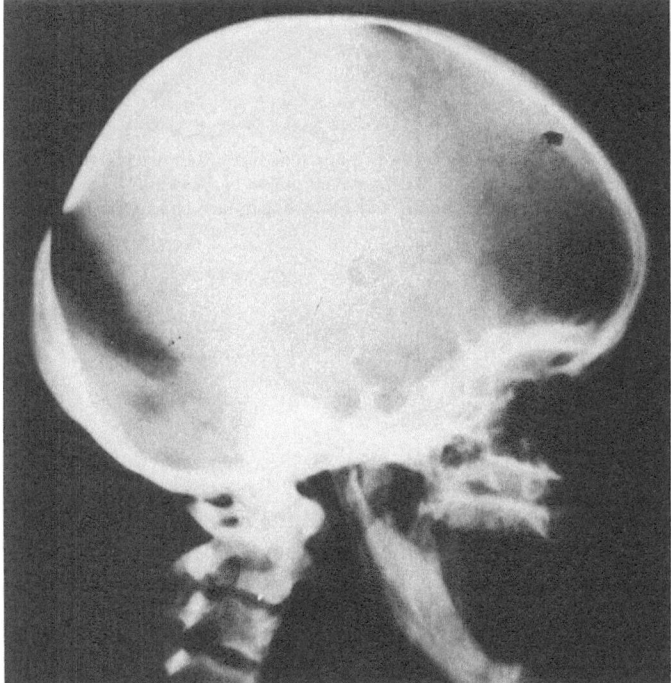

Fig. 8.6. Pycnodysostosis. Lateral view of the skull in a young woman showing an open lambdoid suture, wormian bones, a thin sclerotic calvarium and basal sclerosis. The mandibular angle is obtuse.

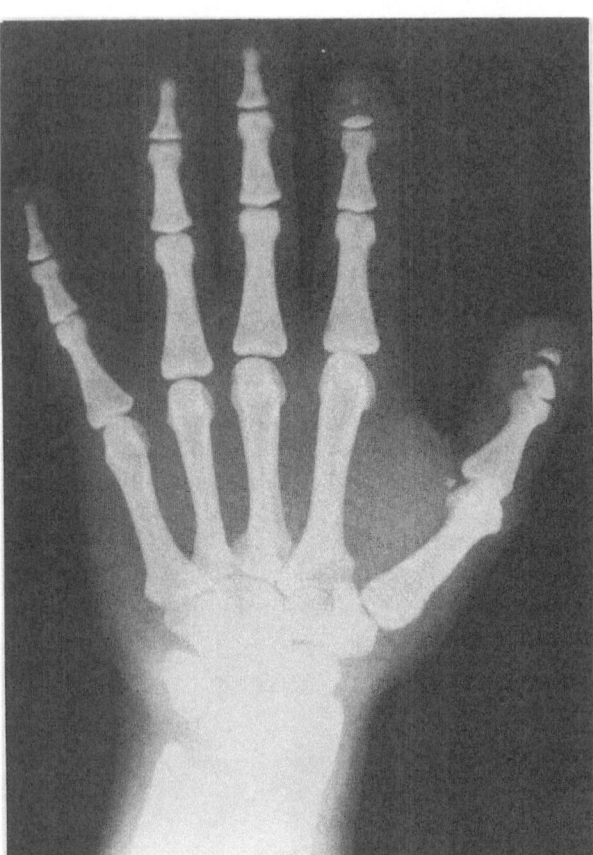 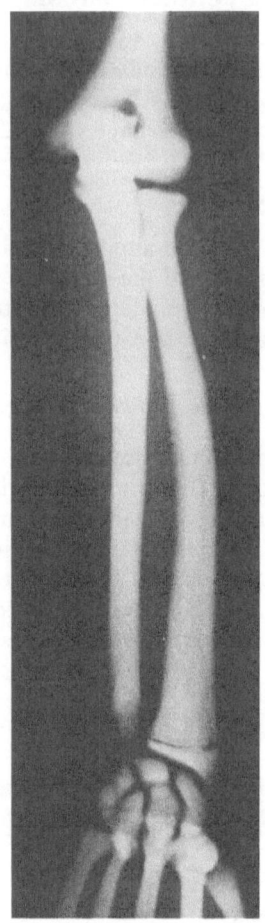

Fig. 8.7. (left) Pycnodysostosis. Radiograph of a hand of the same patient as Fig. 8.6 showing generalised sclerosis but normal modelling in the digital rays, although the distal metaphyses of the radius and ulna are broad. The dysplastic terminal phalanges seen in the thumb and index fingers are characteristic.

Fig. 8.8. (right) Pycnodysostosis. Mild Madelung deformity.

Genetics

Pycnodysostosis is inherited as an autosomal recessive trait.

Management

The disorder may produce surprisingly little disability and the majority of reports of orthopaedic complications concern transverse fractures in the long bones (Fig. 8.9). Some patients have brittle bones and sustain numerous fractures (Elmore 1967; Meredith et al. 1978), but others have few such problems (Roth 1976; Taylor et al. 1978). Most fractures heal without difficulty but delayed union has been reported (Meredith et al. 1978). Internal fixation may be safely undertaken but the hardness of the bone hinders introduction of screws and nails. Teeth extraction may prove difficult and mandibular fractures have been recorded (Elmore 1967).

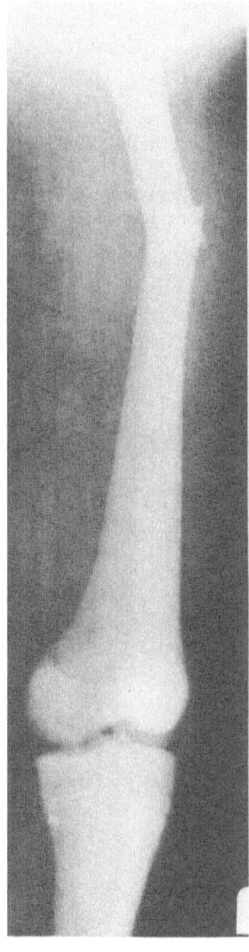

Fig. 8.9. Pycnodysostosis. Transverse fracture in the shaft of the femur.

References

Osteopetrosis

Ballet JP, Griscelli C, Coutris G, Milhard G, Maroteaux P (1977) Bone marrow transplantation in osteopetrosis. Lancet II:1137

Breck LW, Cornell RC, Emmett JE (1975) Intramedullary fixation of fractures of the femur in a case of osteopetrosis. J Bone Joint Surg [Am] 39:1389

Cameron HU, Dewar FP (1977) Degenerative osteoarthritis associated with osteopetrosis. Clin Orthop 127:148

Hamersma H (1970) Osteopetrosis (marble bone disease) of the temporal bone. Laryngoscope 80:1518

Hamersma H (1974) Total decompression of the facial nerve in osteopetrosis (marble bone disease—morbus Albers-Schönberg). J Otorlaryngol 36:21

Mainous EG, Hart GB, Soffa DJ, Graham GA (1975) Hyperbaric oxygen treatment of mandibular osteomyelitis in osteopetrosis. J Oral Surg 33:288

Milhaud G, Labat M-L (1978) Thymus and osteopetrosis. Clin Orthop 135:260

Reeves JD, Huffer WE, August CS, Hathaway WE, Koerper M, Walters CE (1979) The hematopoietic effects of prednisone therapy on four infants with osteopetrosis. J Pediatr 94.2:210

Shapiro F, Glimcher MJ, Holtrop ME, Tashjian AHJ, Brickley-Parsons D, Kenzora J (1980) Human osteopetrosis; a histological, ultrastructural and biochemical study. J Bone Joint Surg [Am] 62:384

Walker DG (1973) Osteopetrosis cured by temporary parabiosis. Science 180:875

Pycnodysostosis

Elmore SM (1967) Pycnodysostosis: a review. J Bone Joint Surg [Am] 49:153
Maroteaux P, Lamy M (1962) La pycnodysostose. Presse Méd 70:999
Maroteaux P, Lamy M (1965) The malady of Toulouse-Lautrec. JAMA 191:715
Meredith SC, Simon MA, Laros GS, Jackson MA (1978) Pycnodysostosis: a clinical, pathological and ultramicroscopic study of a case. J Bone Joint Surg [Am] 60:1122
Roth VG (1976) Pycnodysostosis presenting with bilateral subtrochanteric fractures. Clin Orthop 117:247
Taylor MM, Moore TM, Harvey JP Jr (1978) Pycnodysostosis; a case report. J Bone Joint Surg [Am] 60:1128

9. Craniotubular Dysplasias and Hyperostoses

The craniotubular dysplasias and hyperostoses are a group of disorders in which abnormal skeletal modelling and increased bone density are the principal features.

9.1 Craniometaphyseal Dysplasia

Craniometaphyseal dysplasia (C.M.D.) is the most common disorder in this category.

Clinical Features (Fig. 9.1)

Progressive expansion and thickening of the skull and mandible distort the face and jaw. These changes are very variable in degree and do not worsen after early adulthood. Paranasal bossing is present in infancy and progresses until early adolescence after which it tends to regress. Many patients develop facial palsy and

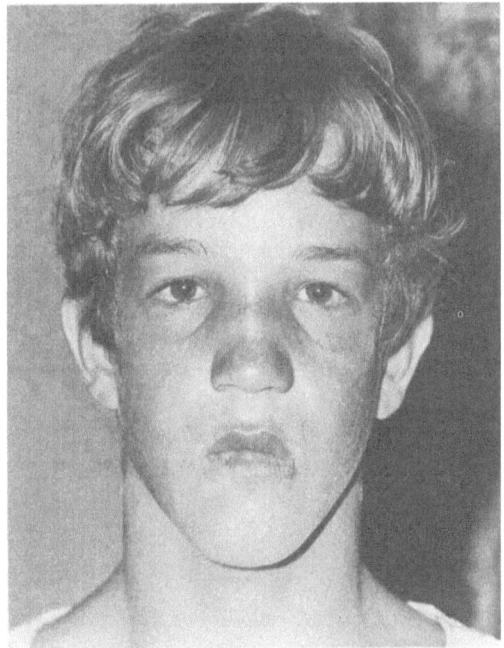

Fig. 9.1. Craniometaphyseal dysplasia. Paranasal bossing in a boy aged 15. From Beighton et al. 1979.

some degree of deafness due to compression of the cranial nerves in the bony foramina. Stature is normal, the bones are not fragile and pathological fractures do not occur.

Radiographic Appearances (Fig. 9.2–9.4)

Radiographic changes are age-related and are usually apparent by the age of five (Spiro et al. 1975). The skull shows progressive sclerosis which may differ in degree within a kindred. The mandible, clavicles and ribs are widened and have abnormal modelling, but the spine and pelvis are normal.

The metaphyses of the tubular bones are broad and undermodelled but do not show undue sclerosis. All the long bones are affected but the changes are particularly evident at the knee, where the lower femur has a club-shaped configuration.

Genetics

The majority of published pedigrees from families with C.M.D. show autosomal dominant transmission (Beighton et al. 1979). In a rare autosomal recessive form of the disorder the stigmata are of much greater severity.

Management

Facial palsy and deafness, which may be the presenting features, require specialist supervision. Dental problems may arise from malocclusion due to jaw asymmetry,

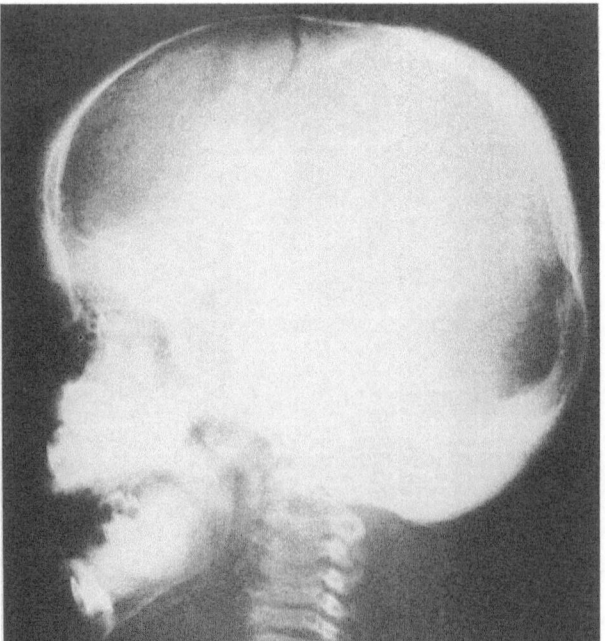

Fig. 9.2. Craniometaphyseal dysplasia. Lateral radiograph of an adult skull showing marked basal sclerosis and thickening of the calvarium.

but early tooth decay does not occur and osteomyelitis of the jaw has not been described. In the patients who have sustained fractures through 'normal' trauma, healing has been uneventful.

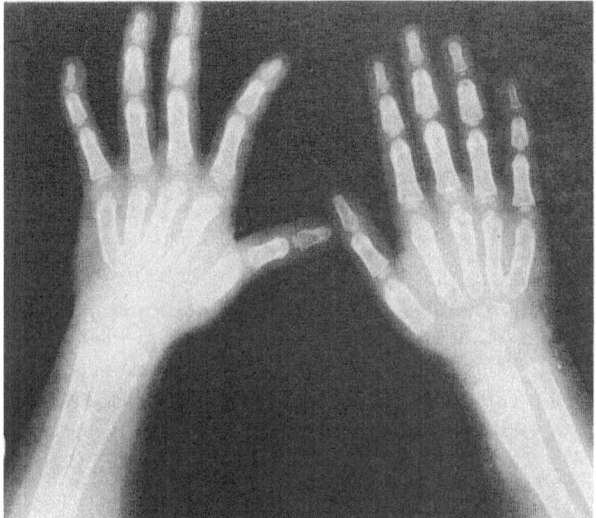

Fig. 9.3. Craniometaphyseal dysplasia. Radiograph of the hands of a child showing broadening of the tubular bones and metaphyseal undermodelling in the forearm.

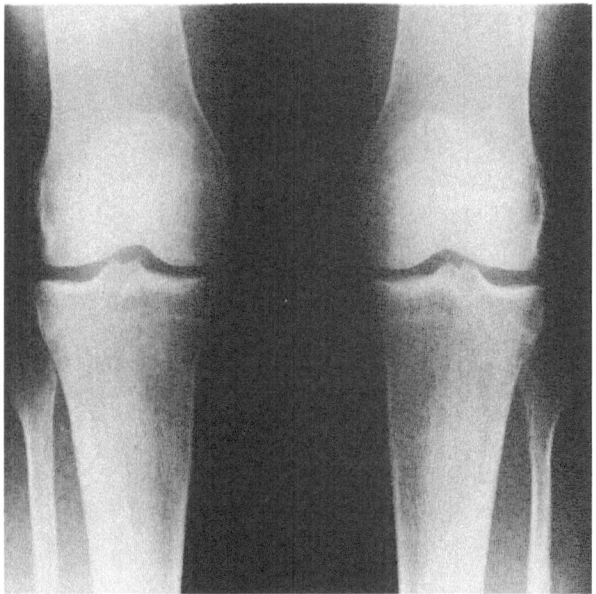

Fig. 9.4. Craniometaphyseal dysplasia. AP view of knees in an adult showing metaphyseal undermodelling but no increase in bone density. From Beighton et al. 1979.

9.2 Metaphyseal Dysplasia (Pyle Disease)

Pyle disease has been the subject of semantic confusion with craniometaphyseal dysplasia but they are separate disorders.

Clinical Features

The only obvious abnormality in metaphyseal dysplasia is the valgus deformity of the knees but there may be minor degrees of limb length disproportion and a mild scoliosis. Bone fragility has been reported in a few patients.

Radiographic Appearances (Fig. 9.5)

The most striking changes are seen in the tubular bones which show gross metaphyseal flaring extending into the diaphyses. All the tubular bones may be affected, but the changes are most marked at the knees where the femora present an extreme 'Erlenmeyer Flask' deformity. The cortices of the long bones are generally rather thin. The bones of the pelvis are expanded as are the ribs and clavicles, and the skull shows mild thickening of the vault and base (Heselson et al. 1979).

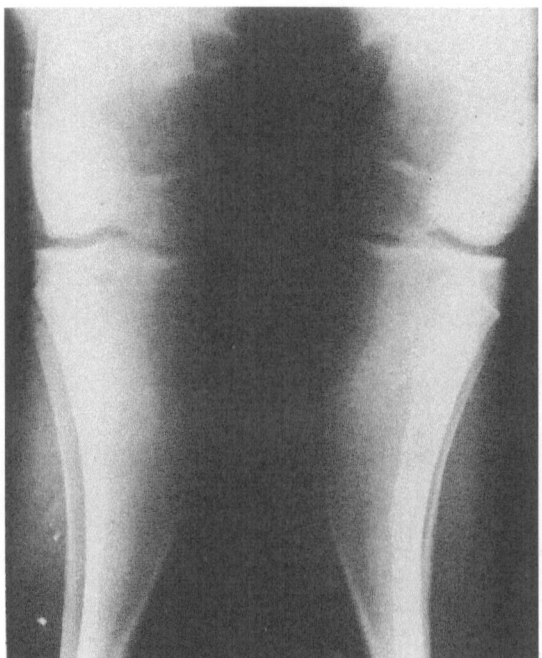

Fig. 9.5. Metaphyseal dysplasia. AP view of knees showing metaphyseal flaring.

Genetics

Pyle disease is inherited as an autosomal recessive and the ostensibly unaffected heterozygote or carrier of the abnormal gene may be recognised by mild undermodelling of the lower femora on radiographic examination (Raad and Beighton 1978).

Management

There is no specific treatment and orthopaedic intervention is not usually necessary.

9.3 Diaphyseal Dysplasia (Camurati-Engelmann)

Clinical Features

The condition presents in childhood with discomfort, weakness and tiredness in the legs. There is a reduction in the muscle mass and the subcutaneous fat, and the gait may be clumsy and wide-based. Occasionally skull involvement produces cranial nerve compression or a raised intracranial pressure. There is a wide variability in the severity of symptoms, but the condition is self-limiting and usually resolves in early adulthood.

Radiographic Appearances

Generalised cortical widening and sclerosis are seen in the shafts of the long bones. These changes are confined to the diaphyses and the metaphyses and epiphyses are spared. The tibia and femur are usually involved and show the most marked changes, but the upper limbs may also be affected. The extremities, spine and pelvis are spared. In the skull widening of the calvarium and basal sclerosis may be encountered.

Genetics

Inheritance is autosomal dominant with marked variability of expression of the phenotype.

Management

There is no specific treatment but Lindstrom (1974) described alleviation of muscle pain and increase in exercise tolerance in a 16-year-old boy treated with corticosteroids.

Van Dalsem et al. (1979) gave a very lucid account of the investigation and management of an adult male with Camurati-Engelmann disease who developed raised intracranial pressure. This description provides an example of the surgical approach to the potentially lethal neurological complications which occasionally develop in disorders of this type.

In the mild forms of diaphyseal dysplasia limb pain may be troublesome (Fallon et al. 1980), but symptomatic treatment is usually successful.

9.4 Infantile Cortical Hyperostosis (Caffey Disease)

This uncommon disorder occurs in infants. The main practical importance lies in its differentiation from other more serious conditions including osteomyelitis, trauma, scurvy, malignant change and congenital syphilis.

Clinical Features

Localised painful swelling is the presenting feature with the mandible, clavicle or a long bone being the usual sites. There may be fever and anorexia with evidence of constitutional disturbance, a raised erythrocyte sedimentation rate and a leucocytosis. The condition resolves slowly and the bony lesions gradually disappear within weeks or months of onset. Finsterbush and Husseini (1979) describe three infants with neurological involvement of a painful limb before the development of cortical hyperostosis. One of these children had an Erb's palsy secondary to hyperostosis of the scapula and the authors mention seven previous reports with apparent neurological deficit.

Radiographic Appearances (Fig. 9.6)

Initially there is slight cortical thickening, usually involving several bones, and this is followed by marked subperiosteal new bone formation. The mandible is primarily affected, but when the long bones are involved the changes are most marked in the shafts, stopping short of the metaphyses (Cremin 1979). The bones may become bowed and increase in length, but the majority eventually resume their original form, although mild distortion or over-growth may persist.

Genetics

It seems unlikely that such a temporary and localised condition could be genetic in origin but there have been reports of familial occurrence which are suggestive of an autosomal dominant mode of inheritance.

Management

Since the disease is self-limiting no specific treatment is indicated, although it has been suggested that corticosteroids may hasten remission.

9.5 Other Craniotubular Disorders

Several other rare disorders are characterised by varying degrees and combinations of skull thickening with hyperostosis and abnormal modelling of long bones. Bony fragility or difficulties in fracture healing have not been encountered.

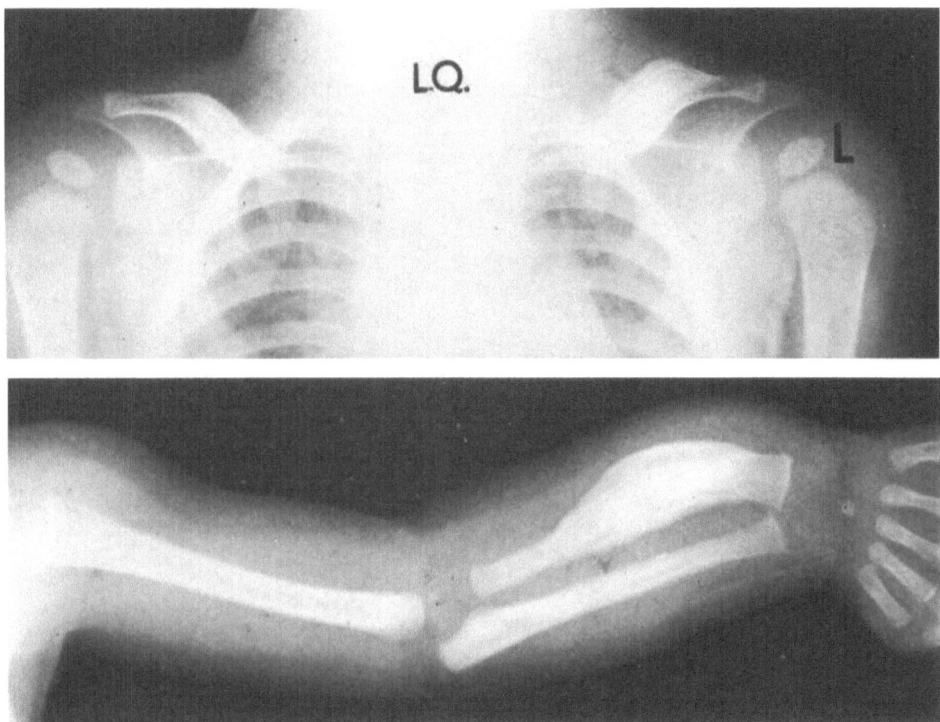

Fig. 9.6. Infantile cortical hyperostosis. Hyperostotic changes in both clavicles and the left radius in a child aged 2 months. By courtesy of Professor B. J. Cremin, Cape Town.

9.5.1 Endosteal Hyperostosis

This disorder has been categorised into the mild autosomal dominant or Worth type and the more severe autosomal recessive Van Buchem variety. The former condition has been encountered in the USA and Britain, while the latter is confined to Holland. The major clinical features are asymmetrical overgrowth of the jaw, facial palsy and deafness. Radiographs show cranial sclerosis and hyperostosis of the diaphyses of the long bones. Apart from their mode of genetic transmission these conditions differ in the severity of the clinical and radiographic changes.

9.5.2 Sclerosteosis (Figs. 9.7 and 9.8)

Severe progressive overgrowth and hyperostosis of the skeleton produces facial distortion and gigantism. Syndactyly of the second and third fingers is usually present. Facial palsy and deafness develop in childhood and adults may experience chronic headaches from raised intracranial pressure, which is potentially lethal and may necessitate cranial decompression.

Sclerosteosis is inherited as an autosomal recessive. More than 40 affected patients have been encountered in South Africa, while isolated reports have emanated from North America and Japan.

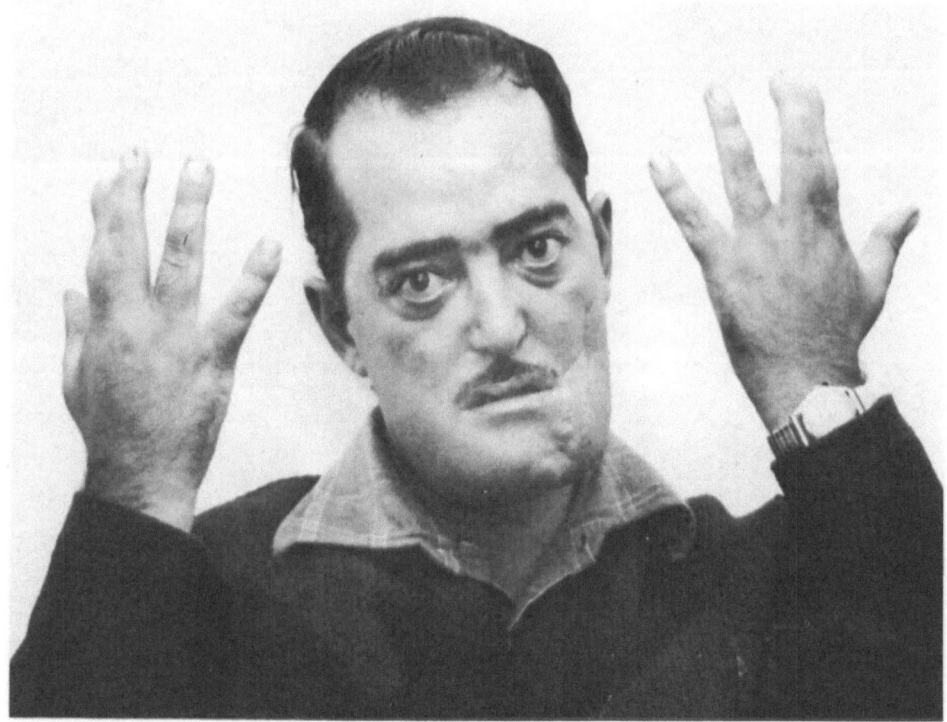

Fig. 9.7. Sclerosteosis. Mild proptosis and overgrowth of the mandible with syndactyly of the index and middle fingers of both hands.

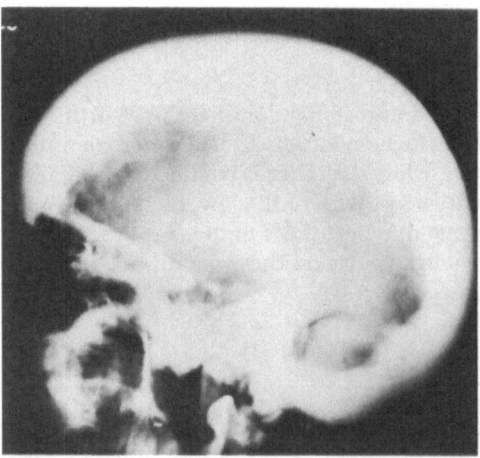

Fig. 9.8. Sclerosteosis. Lateral radiograph of the skull.

9.5.3 Frontometaphyseal Dysplasia

Individuals with frontometaphyseal dysplasia have a visor-like prominence of the brow, hypoplasia of the mandible and mild lengthening of the limbs in relation to the trunk. Compression of the 7th and 8th cranial nerves is the only significant clinical problem.

Radiographs show dense hyperostosis in the frontal region of the skull, while patchy sclerosis in the calvarium may lead to a misdiagnosis of Paget disease. Mild dysplastic changes are present throughout the skeleton.

There is controversy concerning the genetic basis of frontometaphyseal dysplasia and the disorder may be heterogeneous. It has many features in common with another rare inherited skeletal dysplasia, osteodysplasty, and there may be a fundamental link between these conditions.

9.5.4 Craniodiaphyseal Dysplasia

The main characteristics of this rare disorder are gross facial distortion and cranial nerve entrapment. Changes in the skull may be very severe, and the non-specific designation 'Leontiasis Ossium' has been applied in the past. The long bones are straight with absence of the normal metaphyseal flare.

References

Beighton P, Hamersma H, Horan FT (1979) Craniometaphyseal dysplasia—variability of expression within a large kindred. Clin Genet 15:252
Spiro PC, Hamersma H, Beighton P (1975) Radiology of the autosomal dominant form of craniometaphyseal dysplasia. S Afr Med J 49:839

Metaphyseal Dysplasia (Pyle disease)

Heselson NG, Raad MS, Hamersma H, Cremin BJ, Beighton P (1979) The radiological manifestations of metaphyseal dysplasia (Pyle disease). Br J Radiol 52:431
Raad M, Beighton P (1978) Autosomal recessive inheritance of metaphyseal dysplasia (Pyle disease). Clin Genet 14:251

Diaphyseal Dysplasia (Camurati-Engelmann)

Lindstrom JA (1974) Diaphyseal dysplasia (Engelmann). Treated with corticosteroids. Birth Defects 10:504
Van Dalsem VF, Genant HK, Newton TH (1979) Progressive diaphyseal dysplasia: report of a case with thirty-four years of progressive disease. J Bone Joint Surg [Am] 61:596
Fallon MD, Whte MD, Murphy WA (1980) Progressive diaphyseal dysplasia (Engelmann's disease). Report of a sporadic case of the mild form. J Bone Joint Surg [Am] 62:465

Infantile Cortical Hyperostosis

Finsterbush A, Husseini N (1979) Infantile cortical hyperostosis with unusual clinical manifestations. Clin Orthop 144:276
Cremin BJ (1979) Caffey's disease in Cape Town. S Afr Med J 55:377

10. Cranio-Facial Abnormalities

In the preceding chapter skeletal dysplasias which involve both the skull and long bones were discussed. However, there is also a group of syndromes in which major abnormalities are found principally in the cranio-facial skeleton. Classification of these disorders is based on the anatomical pattern of cranio-facial changes and the extent of involvement of the remainder of the skeleton and other systems.

Premature closure of the sutures of the skull results in craniostenosis. The ensuing shape of the skull depends on the sutures involved, the sequence of their closure and the degree of growth in unaffected areas. A misshapen skull may interfere with the growth and development of the brain and the facial appearance may be grotesque. Isolated craniostenosis is usually non-genetic but in about 5% of patients this malformation is inherited. It may be associated with other skeletal and visceral abnormalities in a number of genetic syndromes, and can also be the consequence of intrauterine or perinatal trauma.

A number of descriptive terms have been applied to the various skull shapes observed in craniostenosis. Scaphocephaly describes a boat-shaped or long, narrow skull. Acrocephaly or oxycephaly is the term for a pointed skull. In turricephaly the skull is high, broad, and tower-shaped, while plagiocephaly implies asymmetry of the skull.

Many conditions in which the face and skull are abnormal are not heritable and have therefore been excluded from this discussion. The better-known and recognised inherited cranio-facial dysplasias are reviewed in this chapter.

10.1 Cranio-Facial Dysostosis (Crouzon Syndrome)

Clinical Features (Fig. 10.1)

Craniostenosis, mid-facial hypoplasia, hypertelorism, proptosis, and nasal beaking are the principal features of this syndrome. Dental malocclusion and deafness are common and the proptosis produces a 'frog-like' facies. Mild mental retardation may be present, but there are no other skeletal or visceral changes.

Radiographic Appearances

The malformed skull has a high frontal region. There is premature closure of cranial sutures with shallow orbits, mid-facial hypoplasia and relative mandibular prognathism.

Genetics

Inheritance is autosomal dominant with very variable clinical expression.

Management

Advances in maxillo-facial surgery have made treatment of patients with cranio-facial abnormalities a practical possibility. Early and abnormal closure of the sutures leads to compression of the growing brain and to cranio-facial deformity. Since the weight of the brain increases by 130% in the first 12 months of life early operation is required, if possible within 6 weeks of birth (Mohr et al. 1978). A combination of linear craniectomies with lateral canthal advancement is currently preferred, and this has given good results in the management of craniocerebral disproportion, as well as considerable cosmetic improvement. Later in childhood, forehead advancement and cranio-orbital reconstruction may be undertaken and if necessary maxillary advancement may also be carried out using Le Fort III osteotomies as described by Tessier (1971) (Fig. 10.2).

10.2 Acrocephalosyndactyly (Apert Syndrome)

Apert (1906) described the association of craniostenosis and severe syndactyly and termed the disorder 'Acrocephalosyndactyly". The degree and distribution of

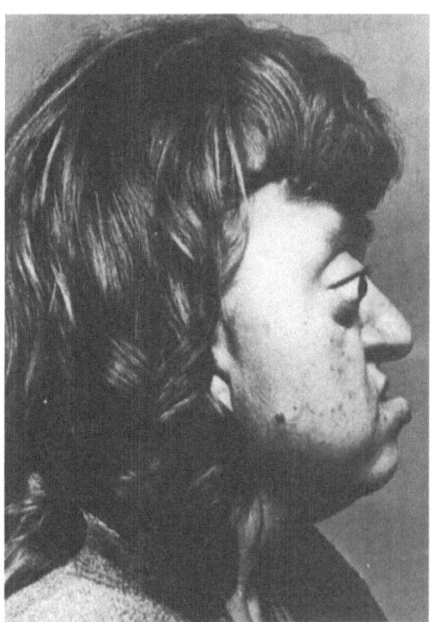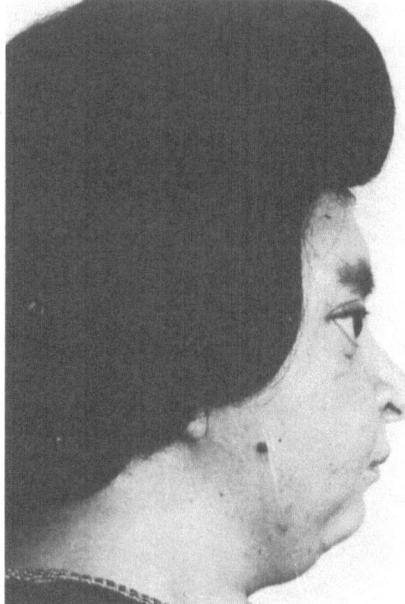

Fig. 10.1. (left) Cranio-facial dysostosis.

Fig. 10.2. (right) The same patient as in Fig. 10.1 after Le Fort III and I osteotomies. Courtesy of Dr Losken of Pietermaritzburg.

syndactyly in the hands and feet and the extent of skull abnormality vary greatly, and at least five sub-groups have been distinguished which bear numerical and eponymous designations.

The acrocephalosyndactyly syndromes are currently the subject of considerable controversy and evidence is accumulating to indicate that they may be reflections of variability in the clinical expression of the same faulty gene, rather than separate genetic entities as previously supposed. The term 'Apert syndrome' or acrocephalosyndactyly type 1 is now reserved for the most common of these disorders, which is described below.

Clinical Features

A patient with the classical Apert syndrome has a high, broad forehead, flat occiput and mid-facial hypoplasia. The hands and feet show osseous and soft tissue syndactyly of the second to fourth digits, with variable involvement of the first and fifth. The appearance is described as a 'sock foot' and 'mitten hand'. There is a high level of infant mortality and mental deficiency is frequent among survivors. The other variants of acrocephalosyndactyly differ in the degree of abnormality of the skull, the pattern of malformation of hands and feet and in the extent of visceral involvement.

Radiographic Appearances (Fig. 10.3)

In the Apert syndrome the skull shows an increase in the vertical height of the calvarium and a decrease in its anteroposterior diameter. The occiput is flat and the

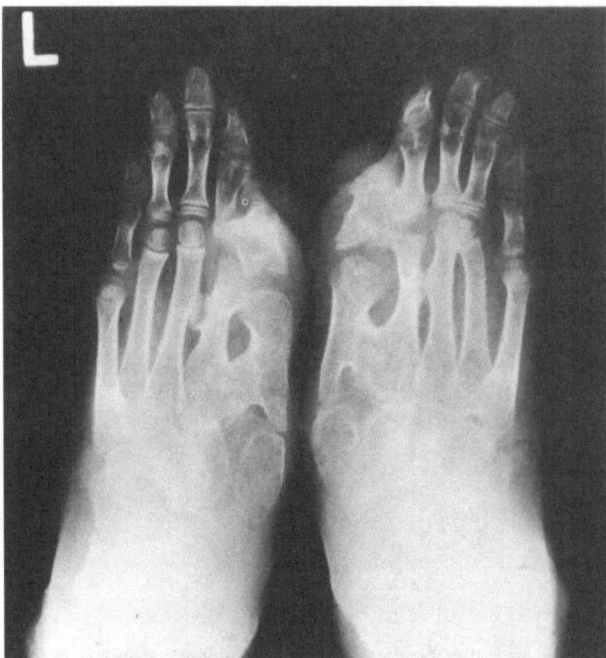

Fig. 10.3. The 'sock foot' in the Apert syndrome.

mid-facial skeleton is hypoplastic. The hands show synostoses of the distal phalanges, particularly of the middle three fingers, and variable metacarpal bridging. The proximal phalanx of the hallux and the thumb is shortened and malformed, resulting in a varus deformity of these digits.

Genetics

The majority of patients with the Apert syndrome have been sporadic, but autosomal dominant inheritance has been demonstrated in some kindreds.

Management

Management involves reconstruction of the hands and attempts at improvement of the architecture of the cranio-facial skeleton. The general management of the multiple syndactylies will be discussed in the section on syndactyly and digital abnormalities, while the current status of cranio-facial surgery was summarised in the previous section. Mohr et al. (1978) emphasised the need for early craniectomy in the Apert syndrome since 62% of their patients were mentally retarded.

10.3 Acrocephalopolysyndactyly (Carpenter Syndrome)

This syndrome is distinguished from the acrocephalosyndactyly group of disorders by the presence of extra digits and structural cardiac malformations.

Clinical Features

There is craniostenosis with a high forehead, mandibular hypoplasia and a flat nasal bridge. The hands show brachydactyly, soft tissue syndactyly of the middle and ring fingers and pre-axial polydactyly, which may also occur in the feet. Mental retardation and obesity are common and cardiac abnormalities are usually present.

Genetics

This uncommon condition is inherited as an autosomal recessive.

Management

The management of cranio-facial abnormality has been previously discussed and that of polydactyly and syndactyly are outlined in Chapter 12.

10.4 Mandibulofacial Dysostosis (Treacher Collins Syndrome)

Clinical Features

Hypoplasia of the zygoma, maxilla and mandible and an anti-mongoloid slope of the eyes give a 'fish-like' facial appearance. Colobomata are present in the lower eyelids and the external ears are small and deformed. Defects of the auditory canals and ossicles lead to conductive deafness. The clinical stigmata vary and the appearance of the mildly affected may approach normality.

Genetics

Inheritance is autosomal dominant with very variable expression.

Management

Early recognition of the deafness enables prompt commencement of treatment. When the hearing deficit is principally due to malformation of the external auditory meatus reconstruction by plastic surgery may result in restoration of hearing, and the facial appearance may be improved by cosmetic surgery.

References

Craniofacial Abnormalities

Apert E (1906) De L'acrocephalocyndactylie. Bull Soc Med Hop Paris 23:1310

Mohr G, Hoffman MD, Munro IR, Hendrick EB, Humphreys RP (1978) Surgical management of unilateral and bilateral coronal craniostenosis: 21 years of experience. Neurosurgery 2:83

Tessier P (1971) Total osteotomy of the middle third of the face for faciostenosis or for sequelae of Le Fort III fractures. Plast Reconstr Surg 48:224

11. Vertebral Anomalies

Abnormalities of vertebral development such as odontoid hypoplasia, hemivertebrae and failure of segmentation are components of a number of bone dysplasias. Of these, the Klippel-Feil syndrome and the spondylocostal dysostoses have vertebral anomalies as a principal feature.

11.1 Klippel-Feil Syndrome

The Klippel-Feil syndrome is probably heterogeneous, and is also a major component of the Wildervanck or cervico-oculo-acoustic syndrome and the Goldenhar syndrome (oculo-auriculovertebral dysplasia). Deafness is the major complication in these latter disorders.

Clinical Features

The neck is short with a low posterior hairline and a limited range of movement. The Sprengel deformity (elevation of the scapula) is present in about 30% of cases, and the neck may also show torticollis and a webbed configuration. Scoliosis and kyphosis occur in patients with involvement of the thoracic spine, while cervical meningo-myelocoele, syringomyelia and spinal dysraphism are sometimes present (Sherk et al. 1974). Renal abnormalities are often found in association with the Klippel-Feil syndrome.

The increase in mechanical stress at the mobile levels of the spine above and below the fused vertebrae may result in severe degenerative change. The consequent instability may produce pain in early adulthood together with evidence of cervical radiculopathy and myelopathy. The atlanto-axial joints are sometimes included in the fusion and patients showing this abnormality have a high incidence of cervical root symptoms (Zimbler and Belkin 1976).

Radiographic Appearances (Figs. 11.1 and 11.2)

Fusion of two or more cervical vertebrae is present and hemi-vertebrae are often evident. Fusions are also seen in the upper and lower thoracic spine and the ribs may show incomplete segmentation and a reduction in number. Dorsal or lumbar scoliosis and kyphosis and the high scapula of the Sprengel deformity are sometimes present.

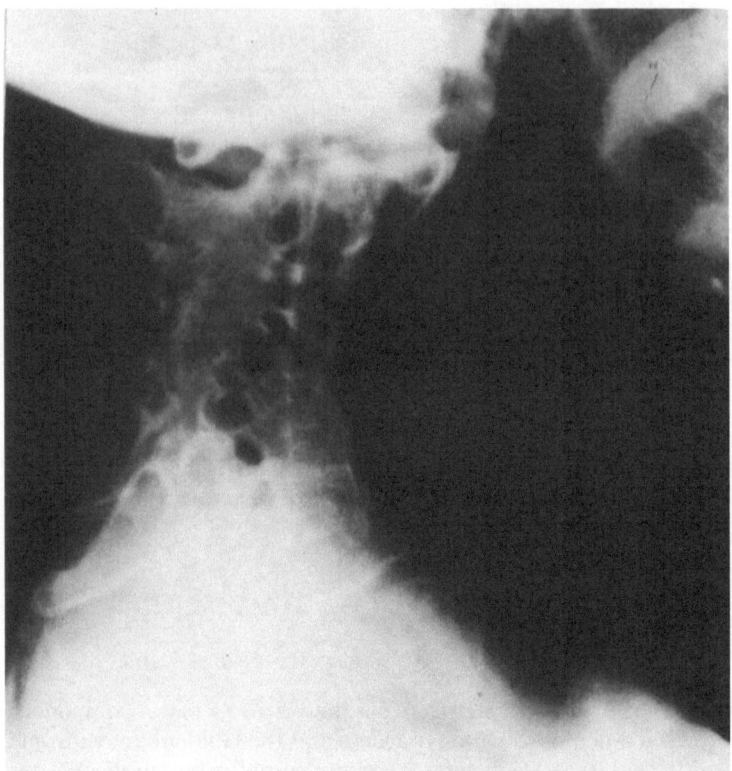

Fig. 11.1. Klippel-Feil syndrome. Lateral radiograph of cervical spine showing almost complete fusion of the cervical spine.

Genetics

The Klippel-Feil syndrome is usually sporadic and non-genetic, but a few kindreds with a dominant pattern of inheritance and very variable clinical expression have been encountered.

Management

Many patients are asymptomatic. Neck and cervical root pain usually responds to treatment with a well-fitting cervical collar, although the occasional patient with unremitting symptoms may require decompression and fusion. Significant kyphosis or scoliosis can usually be managed by a Milwaukee brace but fusion is sometimes necessary. The high incidence of abnormality of the urinary tract warrants routine intravenous pyelography in every patient with the Klippel-Feil syndrome.

11.2 Costovertebral Segmentation Anomalies

The term 'spondylocostal dysostosis' (S.C.D.) was used in the 1977 International Nomenclature for Constitutional Disorders of Bone for syndromes of vertebral

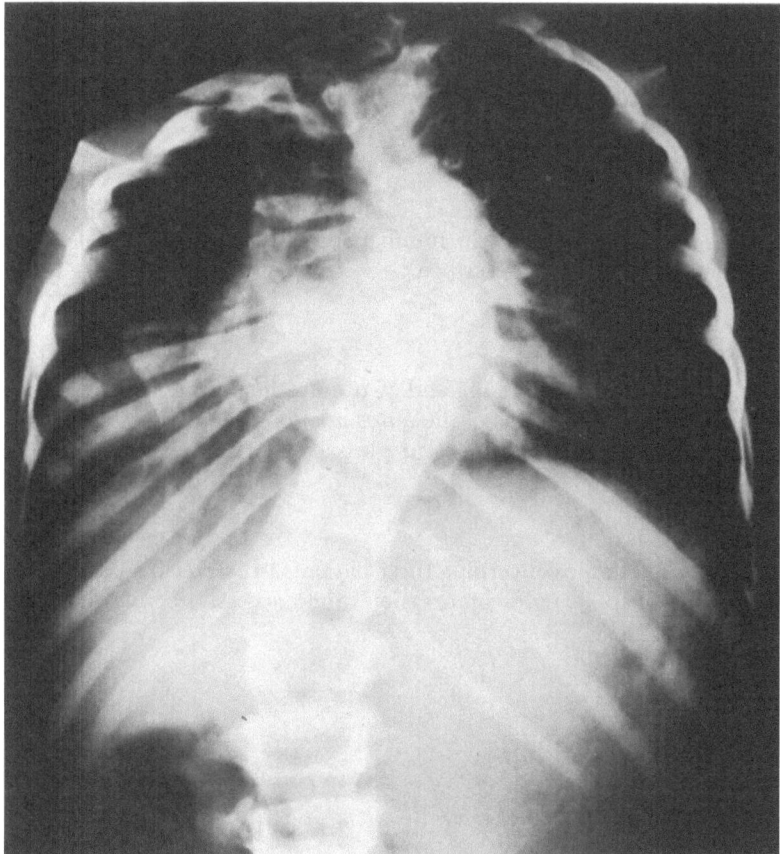

Fig. 11.2. Klippel-Feil syndrome. Associated thoracic abnormality.

maldevelopment and thoracic abnormalities with further subdivision into dominant and recessive forms. More specifically, the designation spondylothoracic dysostosis (S.T.D.) is applicable to disorders with spinal abnormalities and a characteristic fan-like configuration of the ribs without intrinsic costal anomalies, while the term S.C.D. is indicative of structural rib changes, including broadening, bifurcation and fusion. Occipitofacialcervical-thoracic-abdominal-digital dysplasia or the Jarcho-Levin syndrome has been classed as a subgroup of S.T.D. The situation is summarised below:

1) **Spondylothoracic Dysostosis (S.T.D.)**
   Jarcho-Levin syndrome (subgroup)
2) **Spondylocostal Dysostosis (S.C.D.)**
   Autosomal dominant form (Rimoin)
   Autosomal recessive forms.

Clinical Features

The trunk is short with thoracic asymmetry and spinal deformity. The prognosis varies in the different forms of the disorder and there are reports of affected children dying in infancy, although many more record survival into adulthood.

The spinal malalignment may lead to neurological problems and one girl examined by us had been paraplegic from the age of 13, with a sensory deficit below the level of the seventh thoracic nerve. Her younger sister who had a similar, but less severe, kyphoscoliosis had no neurological problems (Beighton and Horan 1981).

Radiographic Appearances (Figs. 11.3 and 11.4)

The thoracic vertebrae show variable degrees of fusion, hemivertebrae and failure of segmentation. The ribs may be deficient in number and fused at different levels. Abnormally tall vertebrae have been described.

Genetics

The subdivision of S.C.D. into a dominant and two autosomal recessive forms is generally accepted. The syndromal status of the autosomal dominant type of S.C.D. is well established, but the recessive varieties are less clearly defined.

Management

Insufficient information is available concerning these patients to establish a pattern of management, but evidence of spinal cord compression would necessitate investigation and operative relief.

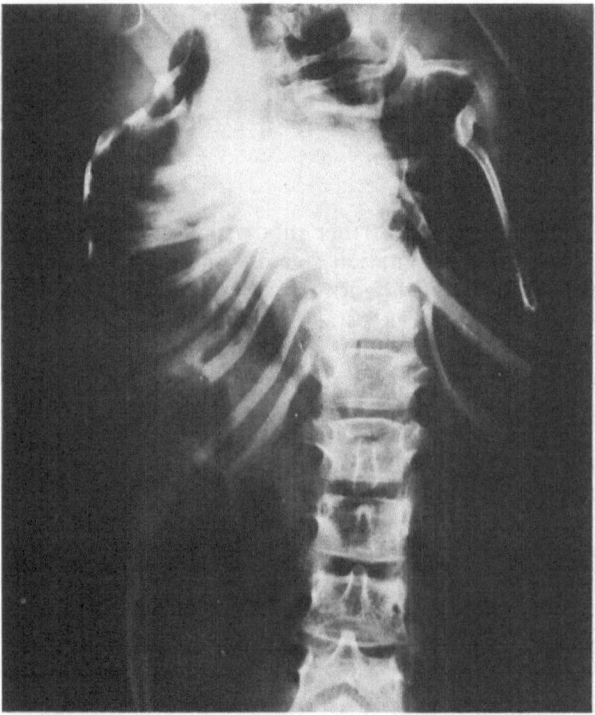

Fig. 11.3. Spondylocostal dysostosis. Marked abnormality of the thoracic spine and multiple rib anomalies. From Beighton and Horan 1981.

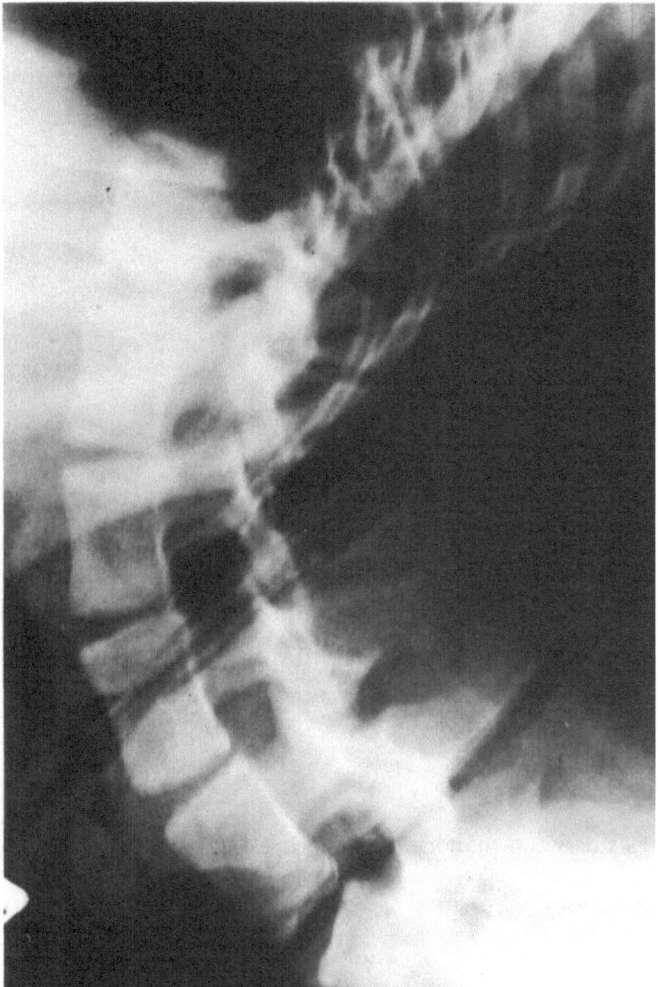

Fig. 11.4. Spondylocostal dysostosis. Abnormally tall lumbar vertebrae.

11.3 Sprengel Deformity

Sprengel shoulder, or congenital elevation of the scapula, may occur as an isolated anomaly, but is often seen in association with other abnormalities of the vertebrae and ribs, especially the Klippel-Feil syndrome.

Clinical Features (Fig. 11.5)

The high position of the scapula throws the affected shoulder and suprascapular region into prominence. The muscles attaching the scapula to the spine and chest wall are often maldeveloped and may be partially defective or replaced by fibrous tissue. In more than one third of patients an omovertebral bone or element extends

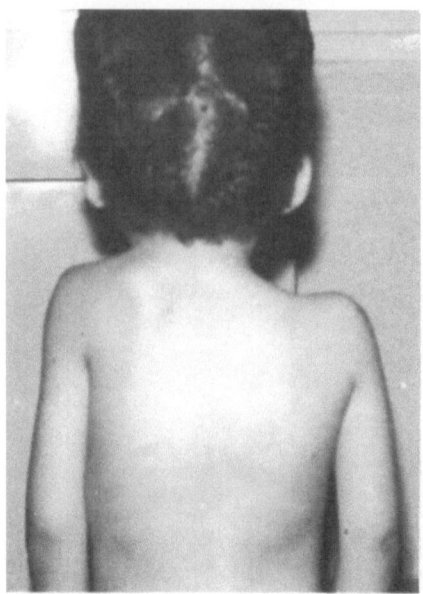

Fig. 11.5. The Sprengel Deformity.

upwards and medially from the vertebral border of the scapula to gain attachment to one of the lower cervical vertebrae. The clavicle on the same side is commonly hypoplastic.

Radiographic Appearances

The scapula lies high and is small and malformed. Associated anomalies of ribs or vertebrae may be evident.

Genetics

The majority of cases are sporadic and do not have a genetic basis but there have been reports of its transmission as a dominant trait in some families (Engel 1943).

Management

The Sprengel deformity may give an unsightly appearance and limit movement of the shoulder, particularly abduction, and the neck. The degree of cosmetic and functional disability is directly related to the height of the scapula and many patients with minor displacement need no treatment. If the deformity is severe enough to warrant operation this should be undertaken as soon after the age of three as possible, since the amount of tissue readjustment required to achieve a satisfactory result rapidly increases thereafter (Woodward 1961).

Earlier operations (Schrock 1926) involved subperiosteal mobilisation of the scapula, excision of the supraspinous portion and relocation of the remainder by fixation to the lower ribs, but these procedures had a high risk of brachial plexus complications, and revascularisation of the scapula remnant, suprascapular reossification and keloid scar formation were reported.

Green (1957) carried out extraperiosteal detachment of the muscles along the medial border of the scapula, resected the supraspinous part with its periosteum and the omovertebral bone, and then moved the scapula inferiorly before reattaching the medial muscles. He reported only one instance of brachial plexus damage in 26 patients who had undergone the procedure.

Woodward (1961) detached the muscles of the medial border of the scapula at their insertion into the spinous processes of the vertebrae in the midline, and released the cervical part of the trapezius. After resection of the suprascapular portion of the scapula with its periosteum and the omovertebral complex, he relocated the scapula inferiorly and held it in position by shortening the lower portion of the trapezius and reattaching the medial muscles at the midline. He noted one temporary brachial plexus lesion in nine cases.

Robinson et al. (1967) appreciated the significance of traction on the clavicle in causing the brachial plexus problems, and advised subperiosteal morcellisation in order to make it pliable and to induce it to reform in a more suitable position. Chung and Farahvar (1976) reported five patients in whom this procedure had been combined with a Woodward operation without complication.

References

Klippel Feil Syndrome

Sherk HH, Shut L, Chung S (1974) Inencephalic deformity of the cervical spine with Klippel-Feil anomalies and congenital elevation of the scapula. J Bone Joint Surg [Am] 56:1254
Zimbler S, Belkin S (1976) Birth defects involving the spine. Orthop Clin North Am 7.2:303

Costovertebral Segmentation Anomalies

Beighton P, Horan FT (1981) Spondylocostal dysostosis in South African sisters. Clin Genet 19:23

Sprengel Deformity

Chung SMK, Farahvar H (1976) Surgery of the clavicle in Sprengel's deformity. Clin Orthop 116:138
Engel D (1943) The etiology of the undescended scapula and related syndromes. J Bone Joint Surg 25:613
Green WT (1957) The surgical correction of congenital elevation of the scapula, Sprengel's deformity; J Bone Joint Surg [Am] 39: 149 (Proceedings of the American Orthopaedic Association)
Robinson AR, Braun RM, Mack P, Zadeck R (1967) The surgical importance of the clavicular component of Sprengel's deformity. J Bone Joint Surg [Am] 49:1471
Schrock RD (1926) Congenital elevation of the scapula. J Bone Joint Surg 8:207
Woodward JW (1961) Congenital elevation of the scapula correction by release and transplantation of muscle origins. J Bone Joint Surg [Am] 43:219

12. Limb and Digital Anomalies

12.1 Limb Reduction

It has been shown in large surveys (Henkel and Willert 1969; Rogala et al. 1974) that congenital absence of a limb or segment of a limb is usually non-genetic, and a detailed review of these anomalies is therefore outside the scope of this book. A concise summary of the present knowledge of these disorders has been given by Lenz (1980).

Radial aplasia or hypoplasia may occur as an isolated defect or as part of a recognised syndrome. The Holt-Oram syndrome, in which abnormalities of the radial side of the hand and forearm are often associated with structural cardiac defects, is the commonest of these disorders. In others defective development of the radius may be associated with a blood dyscrasia. These syndromes have been reviewed by Goldberg and Meyn (1976) who also discussed the management of the limb deformities.

Defects of the ulna and medial side of the hand are uncommon and there is usually no evidence of genetic causation. They may occur in association with malformation of the opposite arm or the legs, and be part of the composite deformity termed the 'femur-fibula-ulna' complex (F.F.U.). Ulnar hypoplasia is occasionally seen with focal dermal hypoplasia.

There have been a few reports of isolated tibial hypoplasia (Russel 1975) but this condition is very rare.

Proximal focal femoral dysgenesis is usually unilateral and sometimes associated with maternal diabetes. Bilateral and symmetrical changes of this type are very uncommon.

Aplasia or partial deficiency of the fibula is usually sporadic but may occur with the ulnar femoral defects mentioned above.

12.2 Synostosis Syndromes

Synostosis, or bone fusion, is most frequently encountered in the tarsus, the carpus and the forearms. Synostoses or coalitions of this type may occur in isolation or as part of well-defined syndromes.

12.2.1 Radioulnar Synostosis (Fig. 12.1)

Radioulnar synostosis usually involves the proximal ends of the bones and distal fusion is very rare. About 60% of reported patients have bilateral changes and the

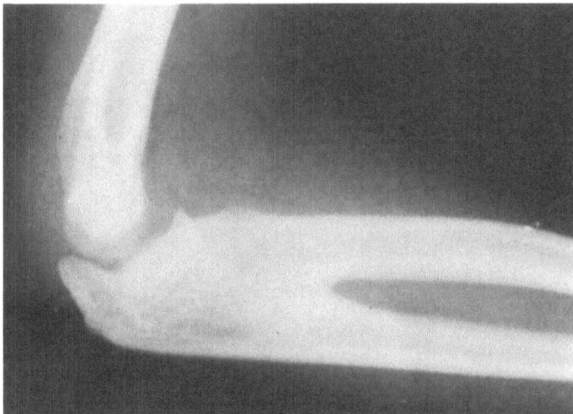

Fig. 12.1. Radioulnar synostosis.

majority have been sporadic, although autosomal dominant inheritance has been recorded in some families.

Radioulnar synostosis may be associated with dislocation of the radial head and may also be a component of a recognised syndrome, such as the Apert and Carpenter syndromes, mandibulofacial dysostosis, diaphyseal aclasia and the foetal alcohol syndrome.

Management

The forearms are fixed in pronation and the radius cannot rotate around the ulna. This position is a considerable handicap, particularly if the condition is bilateral. Early attempts at surgical intervention involved dismantling the synostosis in an attempt to allow rotation, but this proved fruitless, partly because of the associated soft tissue contractures. Kelikian and Doumanion (1957) reported reasonable improvement in function following the implantation of a stainless steel swivel into the upper end of the radius, combining the procedure with muscle transfers to facilitate rotation.

Current practice favours osteotomy through the site of the synostosis and derotation to the position of maximal function, allowing refusion through the osteotomy (Mital 1976).

12.2.2 Humero-radial Synostosis (Fig. 12.2)

Humero-radial synostosis is a rare malformation which may occur alone or as part of a group of anomalies which are usually confined to the upper limbs. The clinical features and the genetics of the syndrome have been reviewed by Hunter et al. (1976).

12.2.3 Tarsal Synostosis (Fig. 12.3)

Tarsal coalition is relatively common and may involve any of the tarsal bones. It is of clinical significance because of its association with spastic flat foot. The common

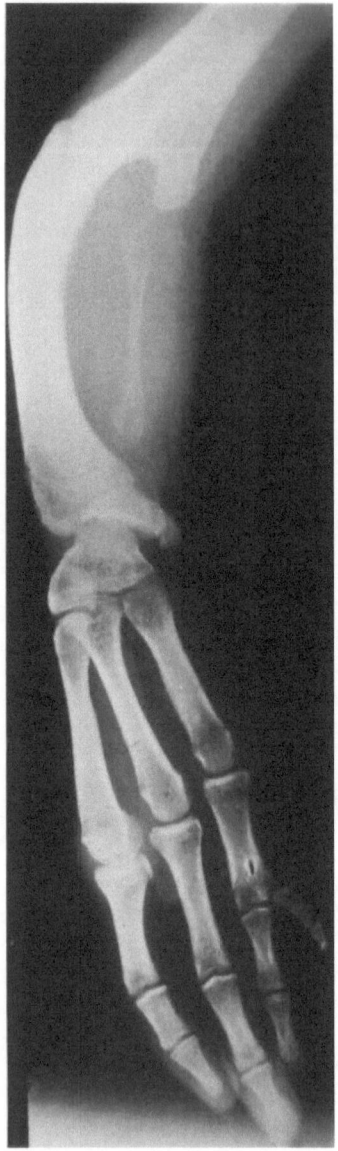

Fig. 12.2. Humero-radial synostosis with absence of first and fifth digital rays.

anomalies are talo-calcaneal and calcaneo-navicular fusions. Leonard (1974) investigated the relationship of tarsal coalition to spastic flat foot and found that these small synostoses appeared to be inherited as an autosomal dominant trait. There was no association with carpal coalition.

Leonard noted that only 25% of individuals in whom tarsal coalition was discovered had foot pain.

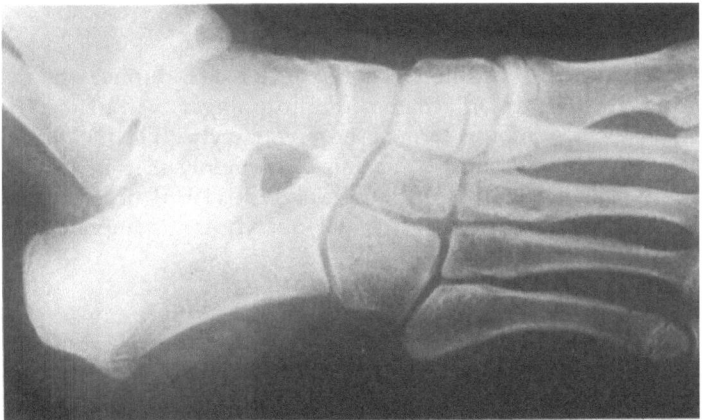

Fig. 12.3. Calcaneo-navicular fusion (Courtesy of Professor S. P. F. Hughes, Edinburgh).

12.3 Digital Anomalies

Digital dysplasia may occur as an isolated defect or as part of a recognised syndrome. The current views on digital malformation have been fully documented by Temtamy and McKusick (1978) in a classic monograph.

This section provides a brief review of the subject which will be discussed under the broad headings of polydactyly, syndactyly, symphalangism, brachydactyly, and ectrodactyly.

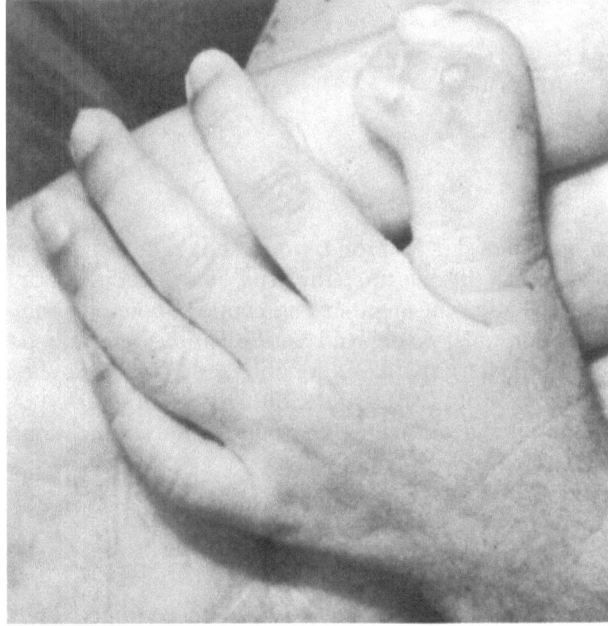

Fig. 12.4. Preaxial polydactyly.

12.3.1 Polydactyly (Figs. 12.4, 12.5)

Polydactyly may be preaxial, when the thumb or great toe are duplicated, or postaxial where an additional digit lies adjacent to the little finger or fifth toe. If digital fusion is also present the condition is termed 'polysyndactyly'. The incidence of polydactyly varies between ethnic groups, being more commonly seen in blacks than whites or orientals (Kelikian 1974). Ruby and Goldbert (1976) described a useful classification and listed syndromes in which polydactyly is a component.

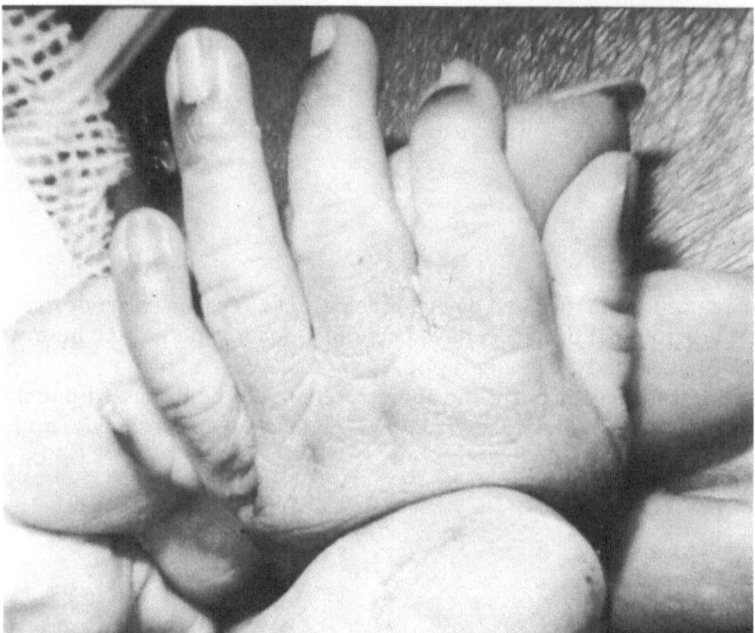

Fig. 12.5. Postaxial polydactyly.

Management

If the additional digit is merely composed of skin and soft tissue it should be excised at an early age (Wassel 1971; Wood 1971). By contrast the true 'extra' digit is not supernumerary but a duplication of the adjacent member and contains bone, tendon and neurovascular structures. Operation must be delayed until it can be determined which of the 'digits' has the best potential for growth and function, and should not be carried out until the child is at least 1 year old (Ruby and Goldberg 1976). The type of procedure undertaken depends upon the particular anatomy of the duplication (Flatt 1971; Wassel 1971; Wood 1971).

12.3.2 Syndactyly (Fig. 12.6)

The term 'syndactyly' denotes bony or soft tissue union of two or more digits. The extent of the abnormality may vary from soft tissue fusion between a pair of digits to

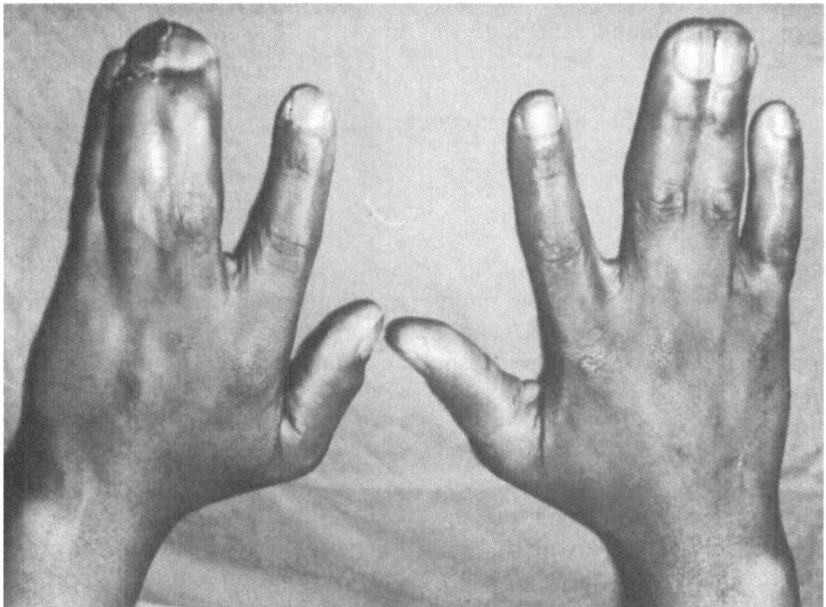

Fig. 12.6. Syndactyly.

complete bony union of the entire hand or foot. Syndactyly may be part of a syndrome or be present as an isolated entity, which may be genetic or non-genetic.

Management of Simple Syndactyly

There are two aims in reconstruction. Firstly, the commisure must be recreated to the optimum depth and covered with the best available skin. Secondly, the digit must be reconstructed and resurfaced so that scarring and contracture are minimised. Operation is best undertaken between the ages of 2 and 4 years, since technical difficulties and the speed of growth make procedures impracticable in the very young, while the child's hand should be as normal as possible by the time schooling begins. Reconstruction of the commisure should be undertaken by using local flaps where possible, and its base must be recessed proximal to the normal commisures, since advancement will occur with age.

In dividing and resurfacing the digits linear scars must be avoided as they tend to hypertrophy and contract. If possible adjacent sides of the digit should be resurfaced with flaps and full thickness skin grafts, although opposing free grafts may be used if necessary. The techniques involved have been described by Zachariae (1955), Bauer et al. (1956) and Flatt (1962), and reviewed by Ruby and Goldberg (1976).

Management of Complex Syndactyly

Basic techniques similar to those described above are employed in the reconstruction of hands afflicted by complex syndactyly, but modifications are required for each individual patient. Hoover et al. (1970) discussed the treatment of the hand in the Apert syndrome and emphasised that where multiple digits are involved both sides of one digit must not be operated upon at the same time. They advised initial separation of the border digits (thumb and little finger) by the age of 1 year. A mobile two or three fingered hand will function better than a stiff, five fingered hand, and ablation of a central digit is often necessary. In such complex reconstruction initial operation should be undertaken when the child is very young so that reasonable hand function can be obtained as soon as possible.

12.3.3 Symphalangism (Fig. 12.7)

In symphalangism some or all of the interphalangeal joints are absent and the digits are stiff. Syndactyly is not usually present. Symphalangism occurs in a few rare genetic syndromes and may be inherited in isolation as an autosomal dominant trait.

12.3.4 Brachydactyly (Fig. 12.8)

The term 'brachydactyly' denotes shortening of single or multiple digits due to maldevelopment of bone. There are many types of brachydactyly which may exist as an isolated entity, in association with other developmental abnormalities or as part of

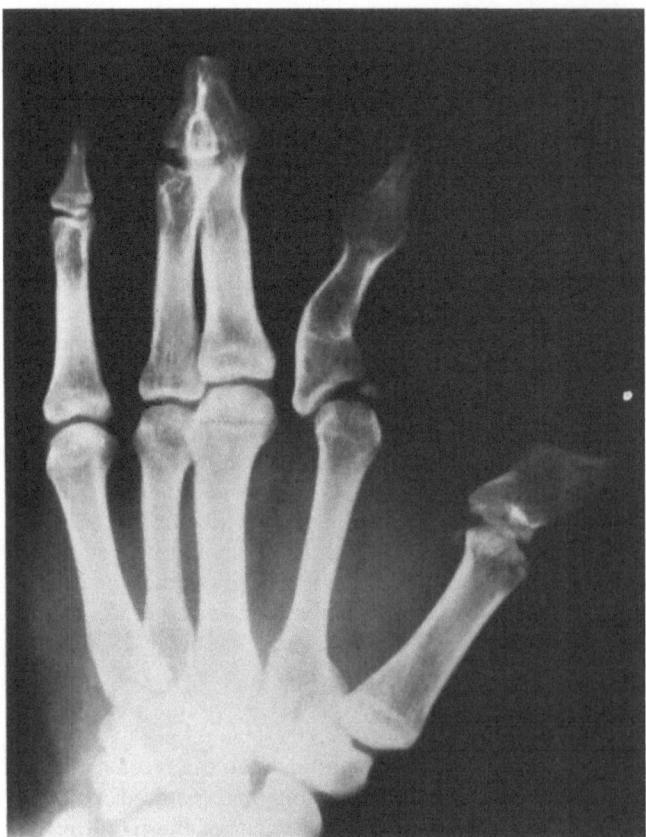

Fig. 12.7. Symphalangism.

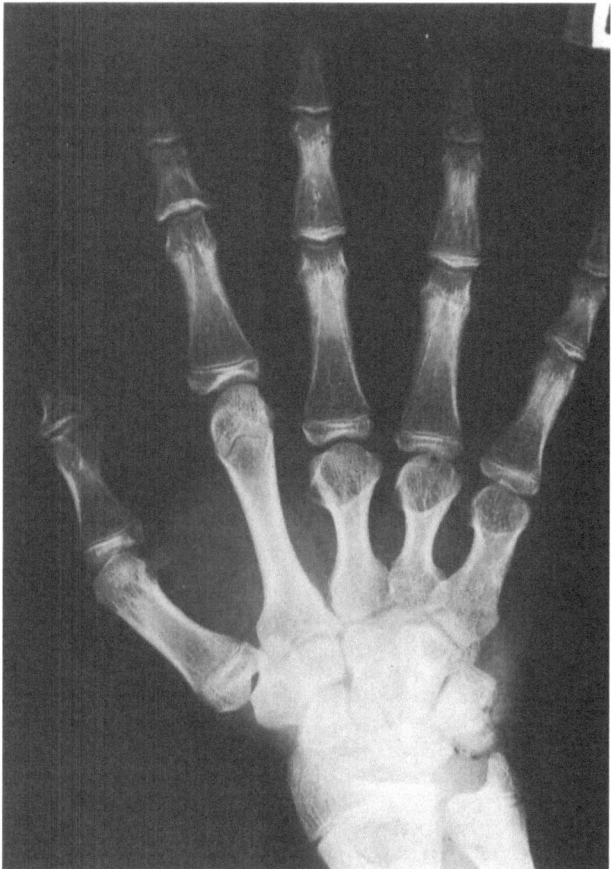

Fig. 12.8. Brachydactyly.

a recognised syndrome. Bell (1951) classified the forms of brachydactyly which had an autosomal dominant inheritance pattern and this grouping was subsequently modified and enlarged by Temtamy and McKusick (1969).

Management

The shortened digits rarely require operative treatment but when combined with more complex hand disabilities they may be involved in reconstructive procedures.

12.3.5 Ectrodactyly (Figs. 12.9, 12.10)

Longitudinal splitting of the hand or foot may be caused by maldevelopment of the central rays of the limb buds, which produces the 'lobster claw' or 'split' configuration. Split hand and foot may be sporadic or inherited as an autosomal dominant or recessive trait. Clinical expression is very variable and a propensity for skipping generations makes genetic counselling difficult (Preus and Fraser 1973).

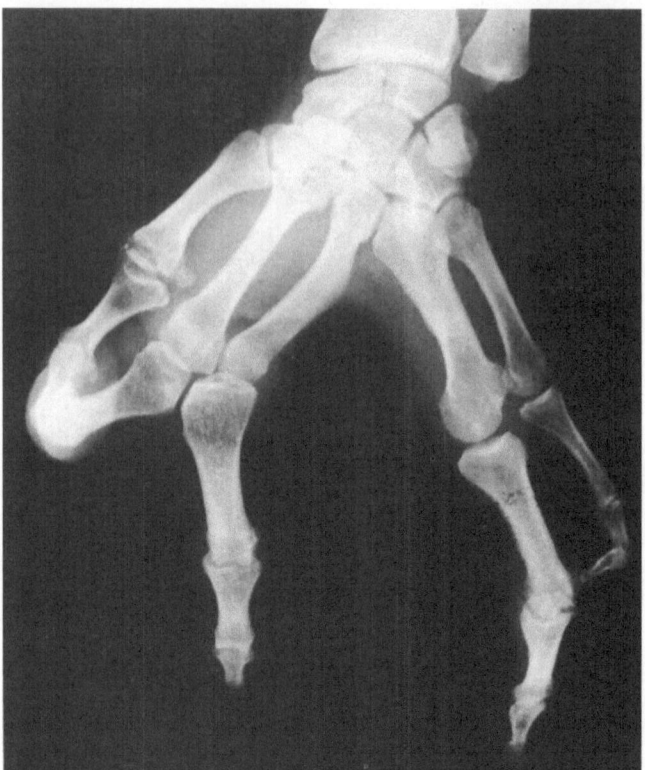

Fig. 12.9. Ectrodactyly, hand.

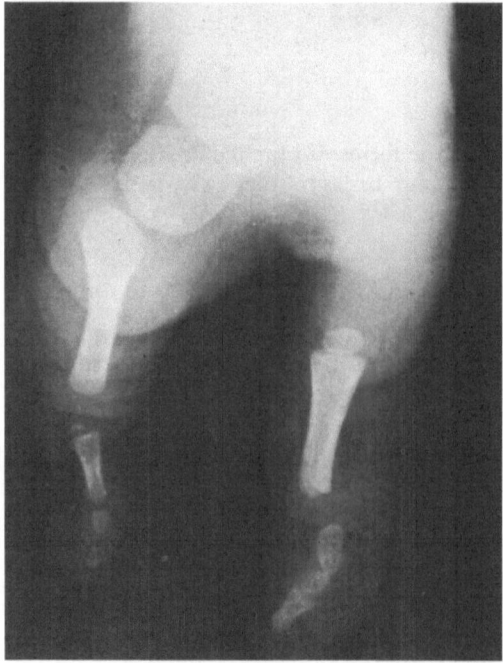

Fig. 12.10. Ectrodactyly, foot.

References

Limb Reduction

Goldberg MJ, Meyn M (1976) The radial clubhand. Orthop Clin North Am 7.2:341
Henkel L, Willert HG (1969) Dysmelia. J Bone Joint Surg [Br] 51:399
Lenz W (1980) Genetics and limb deficiencies. Clin Orthop 148:9
Rogala EJ, Wynne-Davies R, Littlejohn A, Gormley J (1974) Congenital limb anomalies: frequency and aetiological factors. Data from the Edinburgh Register of the Newborn. J Med Genet 11.3:221
Russell JE (1975) Tibial hemimelia: limb deficiency in siblings. Inter-Clinic Information Bulletin 14(7):15

Radioulnar Synostosis

Kelikian M, Doumanian A (1957) Swivel for proximal radio-ulnar synostosis. J Bone Joint Surg [Am] 39:945
Mital MA (1976) Radioulnar synostosis and dislocation of the radial head. Orthop Clin North Am 7:375

Humero-radial Synostosis

Hunter AGW, Cox DW, Rudd NL (1976) The genetics of and associated clinical findings in humero-radial synostosis. Clin Genet 9:470

Tarsal Synostosis

Leonard MA (1974) The inheritance of tarsal coalition and its relationship to spastic flat foot. J Bone Joint Surg [Br] 56:520

Digital Anomalies

Bauer TB, Tondra JM, Trusler HM (1956) Technical modifications in repair of syndactylism. Plast Reconstr Surg 17:385
Bell J (1951) On brachydactyly and symphalangism. Treasury of Human Inheritance 5:1
Flatt A (1962) Treatment of syndactylism. Plast Reconstr Surg 29:336
Flatt A (1971) Problems in polydactyly. In: Cramer LM, Chase RA (eds) Symposium on the hand, vol 3. Mosby, St Louis, pp 150–167
Hoover GH, Flatt AE, Weiss MW (1970) The hand in Apert's syndrome. J Bone Joint Surg [Am] 52:878
Kelikian H (1974) Congenital deformities of the hand and forearm. Saunders, Philadelphia, p 408
Preus M, Fraser FC (1973) The lobster-claw defect with ectodermal defects, cleft lip-palate, tear duct anomaly and renal anomalies. Clin Genet 4:369
Ruby L, Goldberg MJ (1976) Syndactyly and polydactyly. Orthop Clin North Am 7:361
Temtamy S, McKusick VA (1969) Synopsis of hand malformation with particular emphasis on genetic factors. Birth Defects 5:125
Temtamy S, McKusick VA (1978) The genetics of hand malformations. Birth Defects 14:3
Wassel HD (1971) The results of surgery for polydactyly of the thumb. A review. In: Cramer LM, Chase RA (eds) Symposium on the hand, vol 3. Mosby, St Louis, p 150
Wood VE (1971) The treatment of central polydactyly. Clin Orthop 74:196
Zachariae L (1955) Syndactyly. J Bone Joint Surg [Br] 37:356

13. Mucopolysaccharidoses (MPS) and Other Storage Disorders

The mucopolysaccharidoses are the largest of several groups of disorders which are classified as lysosomal storage diseases. Lysosomes are concerned with intracellular degradation of macromolecular compounds into smaller component units. This process is dependent upon specific enzymes, and defective activity of any of these may cause a block in the breakdown process with an accumulation of the semi-degraded compound within the cell. The disorders are classified according to the type of substance which accumulates, hence the designation mucopolysaccharidoses, sphingolipidoses, and gangliosidoses.

In biochemical terms the mucopolysaccharides are usually known as glycosaminoglycans. The three mucopolysaccharides which accumulate in the MPS are dermatan sulphate, heparan sulphate and keratan sulphate, and abnormal quantities of these compounds are excreted in the urine. Analysis of the degradation products present in the urine is of great assistance in recognising the clinical type of any particular MPS. Metabolic studies of cultured skin fibroblasts now allow precise identification of the enzyme defect in most instances, and facilitate diagnostic confirmation. The availability of such methods of investigation has resulted in the delineation of new forms of MPS and the better understanding of previously recognised syndromes.

Clinically the MPS are characterised by varying degrees of facial coarsening, short stature, skeletal dysplasia, corneal clouding, hepatosplenomegaly and intellectual impairment.

The radiographic appearances of most types of MPS are fundamentally similar and Spranger et al. (1974) used the term 'dysostosis multiplex' to embrace the main features. The skull is enlarged with a thick calvarium and a 'J-shaped' pituitary fossa. The ribs are wide and oar-shaped. The vertebrae are ovoid when immature and present an anterior beaked appearance on the lateral view, but become more flattened when maturity is reached. The iliae are flared and the acetabulae are dysplastic. The tubular bones are short with uneven modelling of the diaphyses and metaphyses and epiphyseal irregularity. The skeleton is generally osteoporotic.

The Hurler syndrome (MPS 1-H) and the Hunter syndrome (MPS II) are by far the commonest disorders in this group and are therefore reviewed in this chapter. The Morquio syndrome (MPS IV) is comparatively rare, but in view of its important orthopaedic implications it has been included. The other MPSs are either seldom encountered or do not have orthopaedic complications.

The mucolipidoses are a group of disorders which resemble the mucopolysaccharidoses. They are extremely rare and a detailed consideration is outside the scope of this book.

The sphingolipidoses include Tay-Sachs, Niemann-Pick and Gaucher disease. Significant skeletal involvement occurs in Gaucher disease (see Section 13.4).

13.1 MPS I-H (Hurler Syndrome)

This syndrome was described by Hurler in 1919 and it has been encountered in a wide variety of ethnic groups. The estimated prevalence of MPS I-H in British Columbia is about 1 in 100 000 (Lowry and Rennick 1971).

Clinical Features

Infants with the disorder appear normal at birth and the stigmata are not usually seen until towards the end of the first year of life. Thereafter persistent rhinorrhea, stiff joints, a thoracolumbar kyphosis, chest deformity and abnormal facial features become apparent. By the age of two the coarse facies and large tongue are obvious and hepatosplenomegaly, corneal clouding, dwarfing, cardiac anomalies and joint stiffness, particularly of the fingers, are established. Death results from respiratory or cardiac failure and survival beyond the age of ten is unusual.

Radiographic Appearances

The appearances are of dysostosis multiplex. The skull is normal at 6 months but by the end of the second year the head appears large with scaphocephaly and hypoplasia of the facial skeleton. Dysplastic changes in the vertebral bodies may be seen at the thoracolumbar junction in the first few months of life and a gibbus develops at this site. The combination of acetabular hypoplasia and valgus deformity of the neck of the femur may lead to dislocation of the hip and the femoral capital epiphyses develop late. The oar shape of the ribs is very obvious. The long bones show marked diaphyseal widening, particularly in the upper limbs. The articular surfaces of the lower end of the radius and ulna point towards each other, giving a V-shaped articulation for the carpus. The metacarpals and phalanges are short and stubby.

Genetics

The Hurler syndrome is inherited as an autosomal recessive trait.

Management

Treatment is symptomatic since there is no specific therapy. Plasma infusion has produced temporary benefit but initial enthusiasm for this regime of management has now waned. In view of the poor prognosis orthopaedic intervention is generally unwarranted. Atlanto-axial instability is uncommon in the Hurler syndrome but the onset of spastic paresis has been recorded in a $4\frac{1}{2}$-year-old boy with instability due to odontoid hypoplasia. Recovery followed treatment by a collar, Minerva jacket and eventual operative stabilisation.

13.2 MPS II (Hunter Syndrome)

Charles Hunter described this disorder in two brothers in a communication to the Royal Society of Medicine in 1917. As the condition is X-linked all patients are males.

The incidence is similar to that of the Hurler syndrome and mild and severe forms are recognised.

Clinical Features (Fig. 13.1)

Children with the severe form of MPS II have a similar clinical appearance to those with MPS I-H, but the manifestations are less gross and the progress of the disease is slower. Corneal clouding is not so severe but deafness is common. Hepatomegaly and cardiac valve involvement are present but the degree of mental impairment is less than in MPS I-H. Death usually occurs before adolescence.

In the mild form of MPS II the disease progresses more slowly and the mentality may be normal. Patients usually reach adulthood but are of short stature. Their facial features are moderately coarse, the hands show flexion contractures and the liver and spleen enlarge. Cardiac defects are common and are the usual cause of death, but survival into the sixties has been reported (Di Ferrante et al. 1972).

Radiographic Appearances (Figs. 13.2 and 13.3)

The skeletal changes are those of dysostosis multiplex but are milder than in MPS

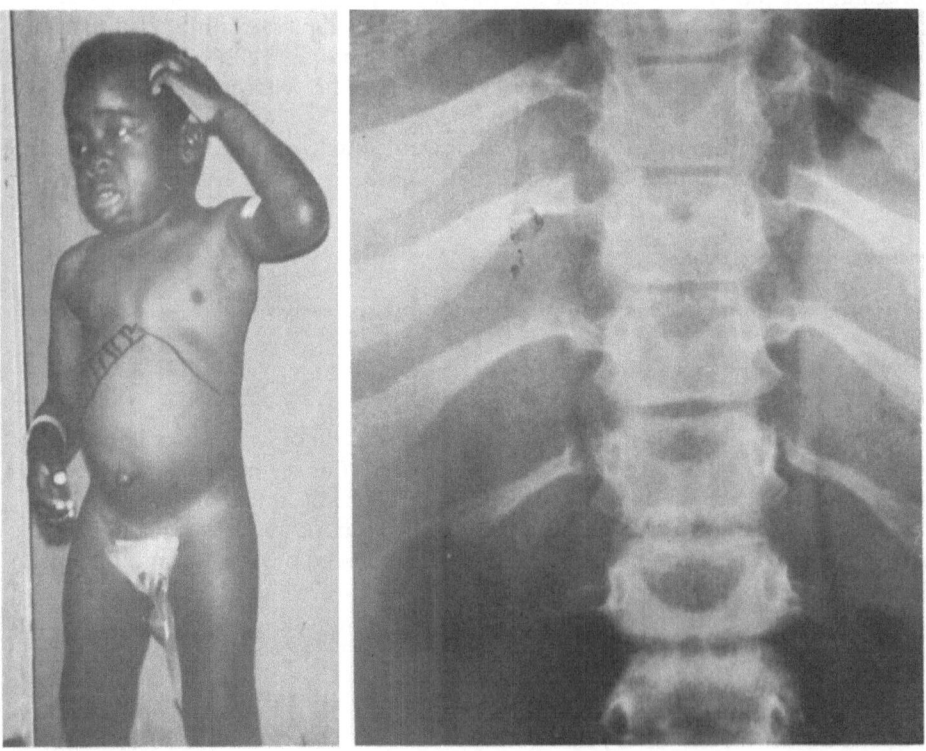

Fig. 13.1. (left) MPS II. This child has the severe form with coarse facies, joint stiffness and hepatomegaly.

Fig. 13.2. (right) MPS II. Mild platyspondyly and oar shaped ribs.

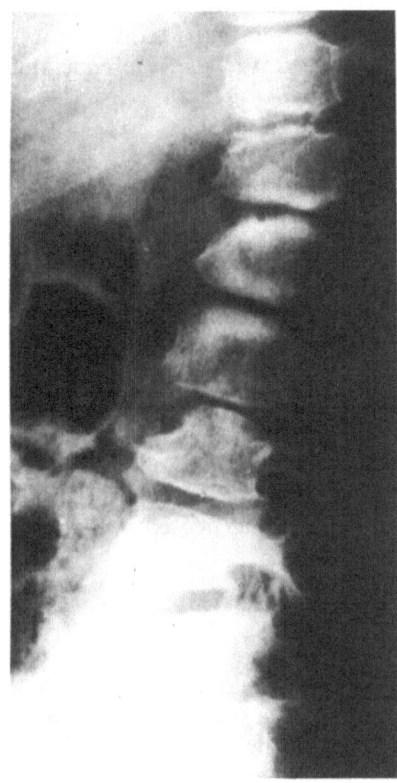

Fig. 13.3. MPS II. Lateral radiograph of lumbar spine shows mild platyspondyly and anterior beaking of the vertebral bodies.

I-H. In particular the vertebral bodies are less dysplastic and a thoracolumbar gibbus is seldom seen.

Genetics

Inheritance is X-linked recessive. The mild and severe forms of the Hunter syndrome were initially regarded as separate entities, but individuals with both types of the disorder have now been recognised within the same kindred. This subdivision is therefore a clinical concept which does not indicate genetic heterogeneity.

Management

Specific problems which require orthopaedic management are uncommon but a carpal tunnel syndrome due to deposition of mucopolysaccharides may necessitate operative decompression.

13.3 MPS IV (Morquio Syndrome)

The Morquio syndrome was described independently in 1929 by Morquio from Montevideo and Brailsford from Birmingham, England. The designation 'Morquio syndrome' has been applied to many patients with syndromes in which dwarfism and kyphoscoliosis are major features. However, in the precise sense, the term Morquio syndrome pertains to MPS IV, and its use in a wider context is to be deplored as this has led to diagnostic confusion.

Clinical Features

Shortness of stature is apparent during the second year of life. Pectus carinatum and genu valgum begin to develop at about 3 years of age and gradually become more severe until skeletal growth ceases. The growth of the spine lags behind that of the limbs. Platyspondyly develops in the thoracic and lumbar regions, but although spinal malalignment is commonly encountered this is seldom severe (Kopits 1976). Odontoid hypoplasia and ligamentous laxity can lead to atlanto-axial instability and cervical cord compression which may produce generalised weakness and signs of long tract involvement.

Marked joint laxity results in instability of the wrists, ankles and elbows. Genu valgum is a consistent feature and mild corneal clouding, deafness and abnormality of the heart valves are usually present by late childhood. Intelligence is normal and there is no coarsening of the facies.

Radiographic Appearances (Figs. 13.4 and 13.5)

In early childhood the vertebrae are ovoid but with ageing marked platyspondyly develops and a central tongue projects from the anterior aspect of the vertebral body. The sternum protrudes markedly and the manubrio-sternal angle may approach 90°. Coxa valga is present with hypoplasia of the femoral capital epiphysis and acetabulum, and the hips are usually dislocated. The bases of the 2nd to 5th metacarpals are pointed and show diaphyseal thickening.

Genetics

The Morquio syndrome is transmitted as an autosomal recessive trait.

Management

The management of the Morquio syndrome has been well reviewed by Kopits (1976). The principal disability results from instability of the atlanto-axial joint with consequent myelopathy of the upper cervical cord. Evidence of this is seen in early childhood with gradual and progressive onset of weakness, even before neurological abnormality is detected on examination. The use of gas myelography-polytomography (Perovic et al. 1973) allows early assessment of cord compression, and reduction of the malalignment and posterior occipitocervical fusion should be undertaken if indicated (Kopits et al. 1972), although the operation presents considerable difficulty.

If atlanto-axial stabilisation has not been carried out the cervical cord is at risk in any patient with the Morquio syndrome. Intubation for general anaesthetic should be undertaken with extreme caution and the neck should not be flexed or extended more than absolutely necessary (Beighton and Craig 1973; Kopits 1976).

Dislocation of the hips does not usually give rise to symptoms. If the genu valgum deformity causes disablement, alignment osteotomies should be undertaken between the ages of 8 and 10, since skeletal growth is not normally marked after that age. Ligamentous laxity of the wrist and ankle may be severe and limit function. Kopits reports invariable failure with attempts at wrist fusion and advises the use of small plastic support splints.

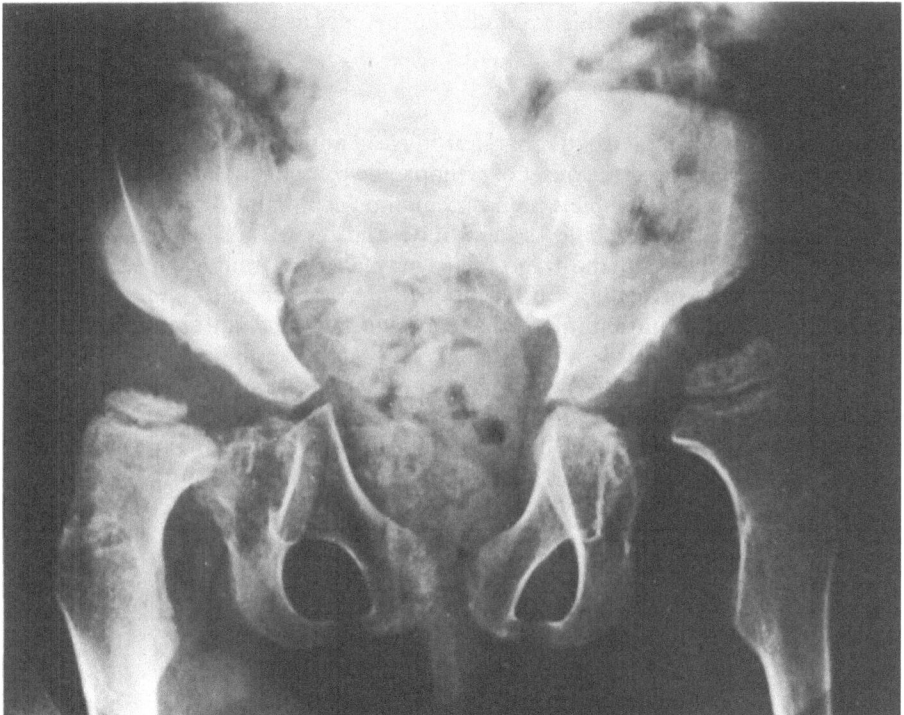

Fig. 13.4. MPS IV. AP view of the pelvis. The hips are dislocated with hypoplasia of the acetabulae and femoral capital epiphyses, and coxa valga.

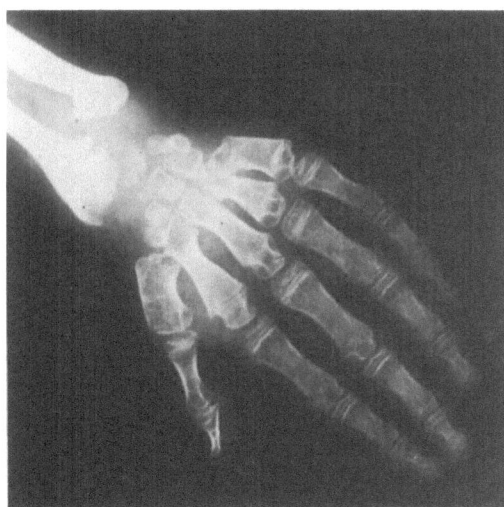

Fig. 13.5. MPS IV. The hands show broadening of the diaphyses of the metacarpals, the bases of the 2nd to the 5th are pointed.

13.4 Gaucher Disease

Infantile, juvenile and adult forms of Gaucher disease are recognised and in each the activity of the enzyme beta-glucosidase is defective. The infantile and juvenile forms are lethal due to the accumulation of cerebrosides in the brain, but the adult or chronic form is non-neuropathic and the life span is relatively unimpaired. Skeletal complications are common in this type of Gaucher disease.

Clinical Features

The non-neuropathic form is usually manifest in early adulthood with splenomegaly or dyshaemopoiesis, although the onset of orthopaedic complications may be the first sign of the disease. Non-specific bone pain is a common complaint. It is usually a dull, persistent thigh ache which lasts for several days and recurs at irregular intervals. Chronic pain and stiffness in the large joints may also be troublesome.

Pseudo-osteomyelitis presents with localised tenderness, redness and swelling, a raised erythrocyte sedimentation rate and a leucocytosis. Blood cultures are negative and the symptoms usually settle after a few days. It may be difficult to distinguish from true pyogenic osteomyelitis, which is also a complication of Gaucher disease (Goldblatt et al. 1978). Aseptic necrosis of the femoral heads is a common and serious complication which leads to pain and limitation of hip movement and gradually increasing disability. Pathological fractures and vertebral body collapse may occur.

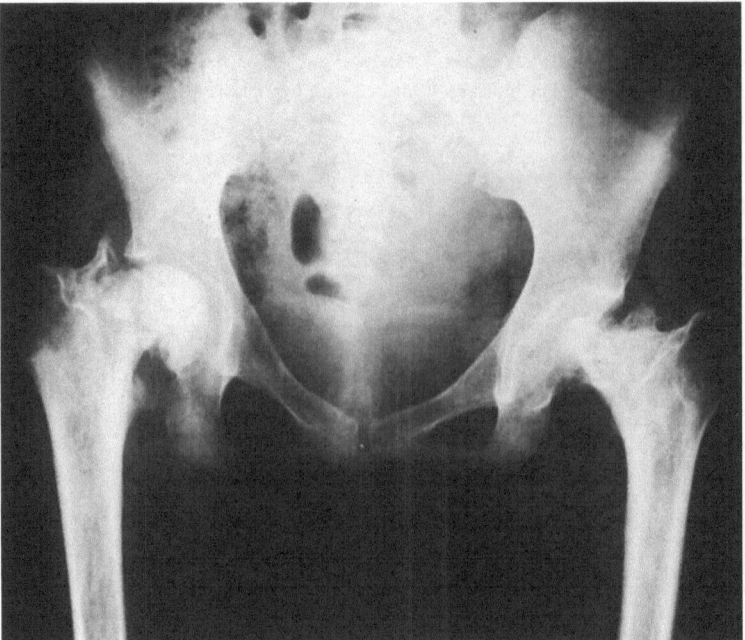

Fig. 13.6. Gaucher disease. Avascular necrosis and collapse of the heads of both femurs with secondary degenerative changes in the hip joints.

Radiographic Appearances (Figs. 13.6–13.9)

Deposits of Gaucher cells produce areas of resorption of bone trabeculae and the skeleton may show a coarse, foamy pattern, widening of the marrow cavity with cortical thinning and areas of periosteal new bone formation. Metaphyseal under-modelling at the lower end of the femur produces an 'Erlenmeyer flask' deformity. Avascular necrosis and collapse of the head of the femur may be seen with secondary degenerative changes in the hip joints.

Genetics

Gaucher disease is inherited as an autosomal recessive. The gene reaches a relatively high frequency in individuals of Ashkenazi Jewish stock.

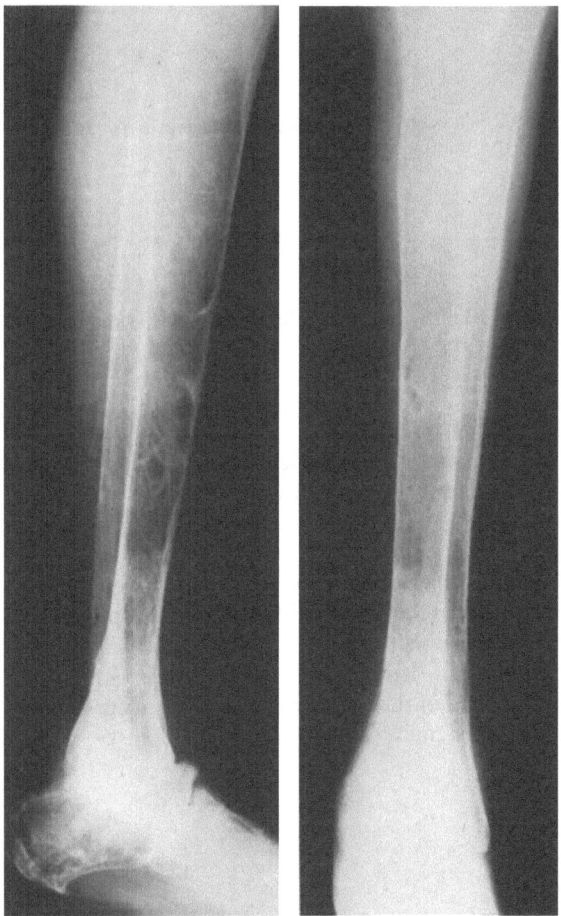

Fig. 13.7. Gaucher disease. Deposits in the left tibia showing the coarse, foamy trabecular pattern, widening of the marrow cavity and cortical thinning.

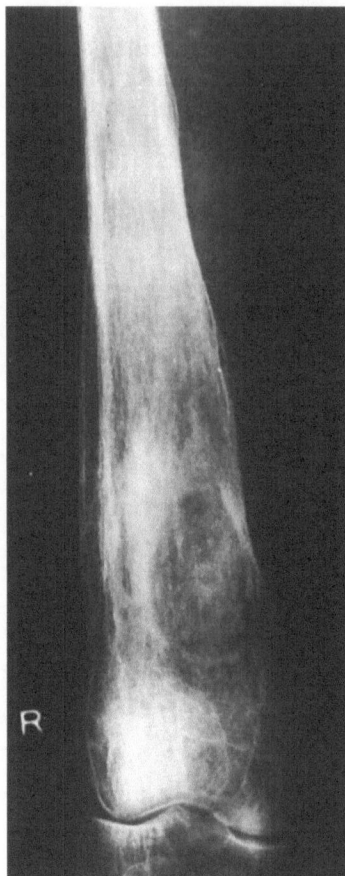

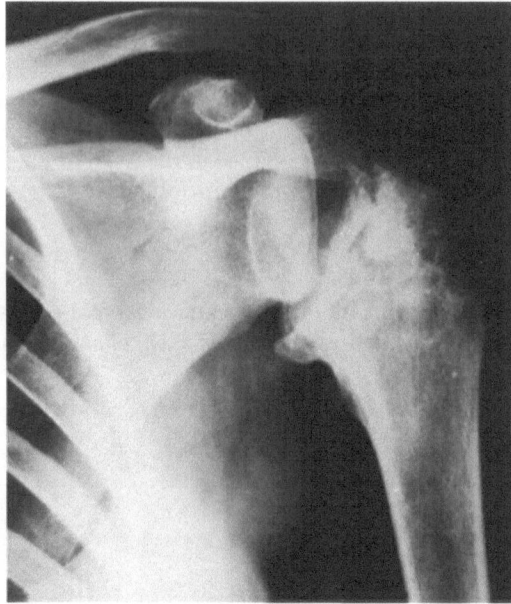

▲
Fig. 13.9. Gaucher disease. Avascular necrosis of the upper end of the humerus.

Fig. 13.8. Gaucher disease. Erlenmeyer flask deformity of the lower femur.

Management

There is as yet no specific treatment for Gaucher disease. Splenectomy often improves the haematological status and although it has been claimed that the skeletal problems worsen after this operation (Schein and Arken 1973), Goldblatt et al. (1978) found no such effect in 17 patients.

Bone and joint pains are usually controllable by rest and simple analgesics. Attacks of pseudo-osteomyelitis are managed by bedrest, pain relief and prophylactic antibiotics. The temptation to aspirate the lesions should be resisted because of the possibility of the precipitation of true pyogenic osteomyelitis by secondary infection (Yossipovitch et al. 1965). Collapse of the head of the femur may require its prosthetic replacement but if arthritic changes are present in the hip joint arthroplasty of the entire joint will be needed.

References

The Mucopolysaccharidoses

Beighton P, Craig J (1973) Atlanto-axial subluxation in the Morquio syndrome. J Bone Joint Surg [Br] 55:478
Di Ferrante N, Nichols BL (1972) A case of the Hunter syndrome with progeny. Johns Hopkins Med 130:225
Kopits SE, Perovic MN, McKusick VA, Robinson RA, Bailey JA (1972) Congenital atlantoaxial dislocations in various forms of dwarfism. J Bone Joint Surg [Am] 54:1349
Kopits SE (1976) Orthopaedic complications of dwarfism. Clin Orthop 114:153
Lowry RB, Renwick SHG (1971) The relative frequency of the Hurler and Hunter syndromes. N Engl J Med 284:221
Perovic MN, Kopits SE, Thompson RC (1973) Radiological evaluation of the spinal canal in congenital atlanto-axial dislocation. Radiology 109:713
Spranger JW, Langer LO, Wiedemann HR (1974) In, Bone dysplasias. An atlas of constitutional disorders of skeletal development, Gustav Fischer, Stuttgart, p 143

Gaucher Disease

Goldblatt J, Sacks S, Beighton P (1978) The orthopaedic aspects of Gaucher disease. Clin Orthop 137:208
Schein AJ, Arkin AM (1973) The classic: hip joint involvement in Gaucher disease. Clin Orthop 90:4
Yossipovitch ZH, Herman G, Makin M (1965) Aseptic osteomyelitis in Gaucher's disease. Isr J Med Sci 1:531

14. Abnormalities of Cartilage and Fibrous Tissue

Abnormal development of cartilage and fibrous tissue leads to significant orthopaedic complications in a number of conditions which are reviewed in this chapter. These disorders are not all genetic but we consider that their inclusion is warranted in view of their clinical interrelationship and orthopaedic importance.

14.1 Diaphyseal Aclasia

The term 'diaphyseal aclasia' was introduced by Keith in 1919 to describe a condition in which numerous exostoses arise from the growth plates, usually of the long bones, but occasionally from the scapulae and pelvis and rarely from the vertebrae or skull. The alternative designation 'multiple exostoses' is sometimes employed.

Clinical Features

The exostoses vary greatly in number between affected patients. They begin to form in early childhood and may be apparent clinically by the age of five. In the long bones they migrate towards the diaphyses but on exploration they are found to have a stalk which runs towards their point of origin in the growth plate. As they are capped with cartilage the exostoses may be larger clinically than is apparent upon radiographic examination.

The exostoses usually cause little harm but they sometimes interfere with normal enchondral growth, resulting in limb deformity. Involvement of the upper end of the femur usually produces a valgus and anteversion deformity of the neck. Vertebral exostoses may give rise to symptoms from compression of the spinal cord or nerve roots, while pituitary dysfunction from a lesion in the sella turcica has been reported (Clark and Attwood 1907). Problems may arise from mechanical pressure of an exostosis upon adjacent nerves or vessels and occasionally the movement of a tendon may be impaired. The exostoses continue to enlarge until skeletal growth ceases. Barnes and Catto (1960) reported that between 5 and 10% of patients with diaphyseal aclasia developed chondrosarcoma in relation to a lesion, particularly in the pelvis or scapula.

Radiographic Appearances

The usual appearance is of exostoses protruding from the juxta-epiphyseal region, the metaphyses or adjacent diaphyses and pointing away from the epiphyses (Figs. 14.1

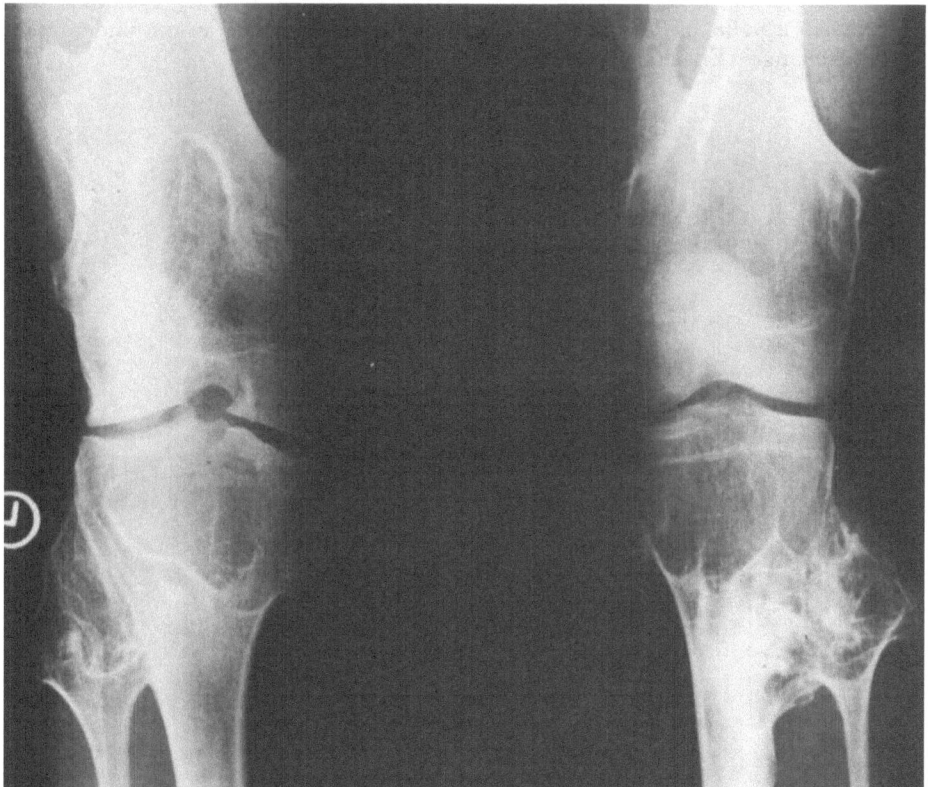

Fig. 14.1. Diaphyseal aclasia around the knee joint.

and 14.2). Irregular expansion of the metaphyses may produce secondary deformities of the tubular bones. In particular the ulna may be short and the radius bowed with ulnar deviation of the wrist; shortening of the fibula may occur with valgus deformity of the hindfoot, and radioulnar and tibiofibular synostoses are seen. Some outgrowths expand and produce a nodulated osteochondroma.

Genetics

Diaphyseal aclasia is transmitted as an autosomal dominant with variable clinical expression.

Management

Individual exostoses do not require removal unless they are causing mechanical problems. Rarely, exostoses developing from vertebrae compress the spinal cord. Roman (1978) reviewed the literature and found details of 22 such cases which had been reported up to that time. Decompression by operation had usually given satisfactory relief of symptoms.

Rapid increase in the size of an exostosis or the appearance of a new swelling after skeletal maturity has been reached warrants operative removal of the lesion because of the possibility of malignancy. When a chondrosarcoma does develop the extent of surgical ablation will depend upon the site of the lesion.

Bone scans using ^{99m}Tc diphosphonate have been used to monitor exostoses and an increased uptake of this isotope has been observed in a lesion undergoing malignant change (Epstein and Levin 1978).

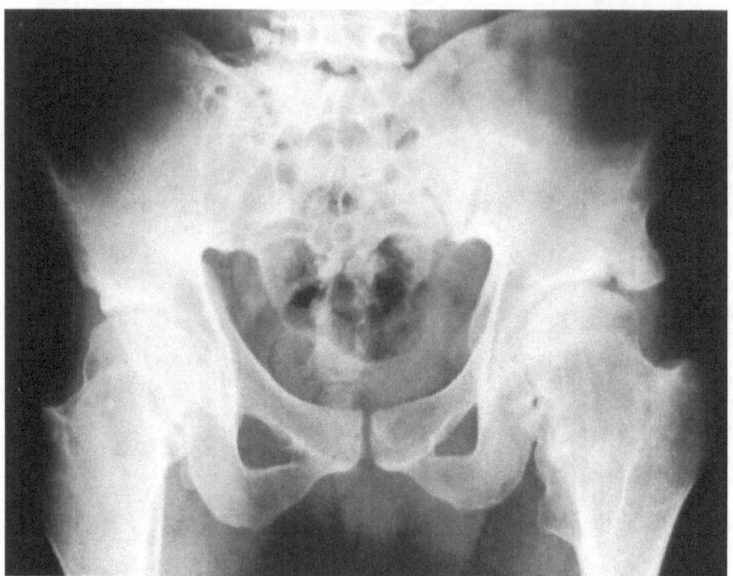

Fig. 14.2. Diaphyseal aclasia: around the hip joint. The neck of the femur is broad and valgus.

14.2 Enchondromatosis (Ollier Disease)

This uncommon disorder is characterised by aggregation of unossified cartilage in the metaphyses of the long bones.

Clinical Features

The metaphyseal swellings may be confined to a single bone, the bones on one side of the body, or, rarely, be generalised. The fingers, the lower ends of the radius and ulna and the knees are the most common sites affected. Lesions of the phalanges may produce gross swellings of the fingers, with consequent loss of function (Fig. 14.3). Asymmetrical limb shortening sometimes occurs and varus or valgus deformities of the knee may arise due to interference with normal growth.

Enchondromatosis in conjunction with multiple haemangiomata of the soft tissues comprises the Maffucci syndrome. Chondrosarcoma has been reported only rarely in association with Ollier disease, but in the Maffucci syndrome the incidence of malignancy lies between 15% and 20% (Elmore and Cantrill 1966; Lewis and Ketchem 1973).

Radiographic Appearances

Irregular translucent areas are present in the metaphyses of the tubular bones. These enlarge and migrate into the diaphyses as growth continues and the cortex becomes

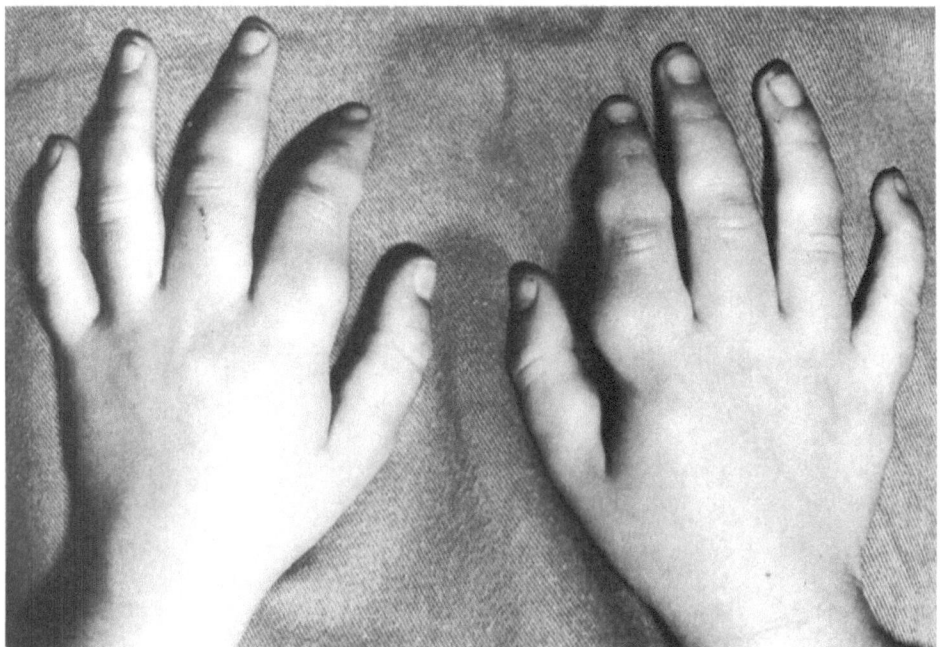

Fig. 14.3. Enchondromatosis: multiple involvement of the digits.

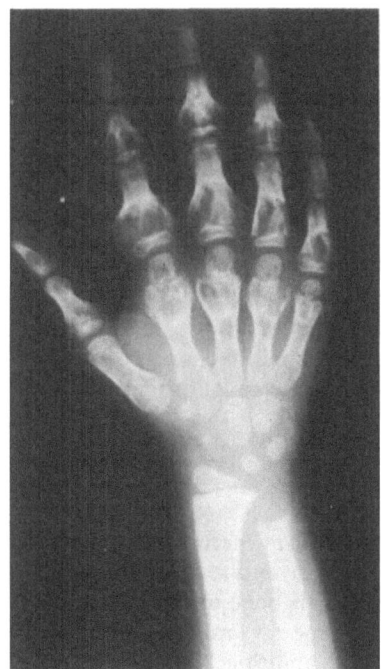

Fig. 14.4. Enchondromatosis: radiograph of an affected hand.

thin and expanded (Figs. 14.4 and 14.5). Progression into the diaphyses may give the appearance of irregular elongated translucent columns and similar changes may be seen in the pelvis. In the hand the metacarpals and phalanges may be considerably widened and a fracture of the fragile cortex is sometimes visible.

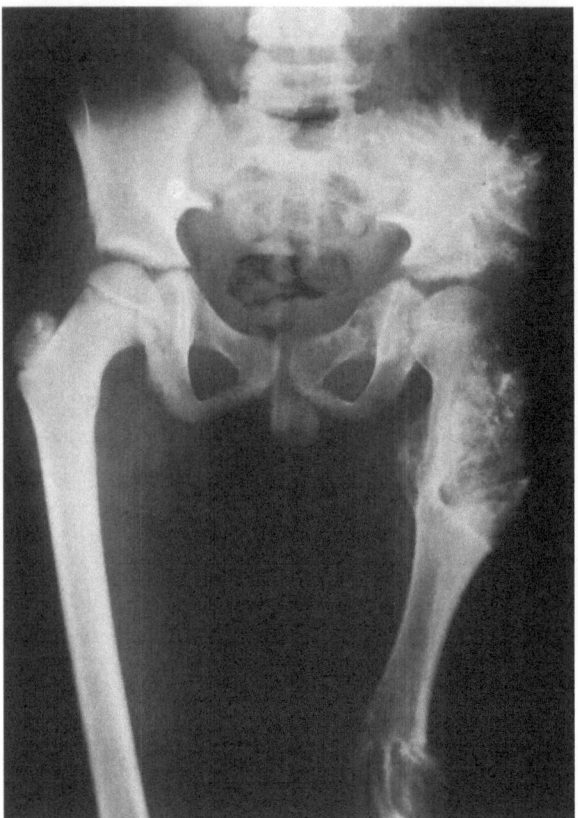

Fig. 14.5. Enchondromatosis: involvement of hemipelvis and femur. The characteristic cartilage columns are apparent. The femur is short.

Genetics

The classic form of Ollier disease is non-genetic but the enchondral changes may also be a component of a few rare inherited syndromes, such as metachondromatosis and spondylo-chondrodysplasia.

Management

The metacarpals and phalanges are the site of most problems. Fractures which occur through the weakened bones are usually treatable by conventional methods. Expanded tumours may be trimmed, curetted and filled with bone grafts (Giannikas 1966). If a number of digits are involved amputation of some rays may be required to facilitate function. Mosher (1976) described a child with multiple lesions involving three rays in one hand which were the sites of spontaneous fractures. He treated eight of the metacarpals and phalanges by sub-total, subperiosteal diaphysesectomy, with replacement of the diaphyses by fibular cortical struts or, in the smallest lesions, iliac cancellous bone chips. An excellent functional and radiographic result was obtained. Takigawa (1971) reviewed 110 cases of chondromata of bones of the hand, including many examples of multiple enchondromatosis.

Lower limb shortening may be severe and leg equalisation by epiphyseal arrest or lengthening procedures is sometimes necessary.

14.3 Neurofibromatosis (Von Recklinghausen Disease)

Neurofibromatosis is one of the best-known genetic disorders and has excited the interest of generations of students, while the numerous and diverse complications have taxed the clinical ingenuity of their teachers.

Clinical Features

The clinical features are extremely variable. Cutaneous manifestations range from the café-au-lait spots, which first appear in infancy, to widespread pedunculated and sessile dermal tumours, which are not usually encountered until later in childhood (Fig. 14.6). Plexiform neuromata may develop into pendulous dermal lesions.

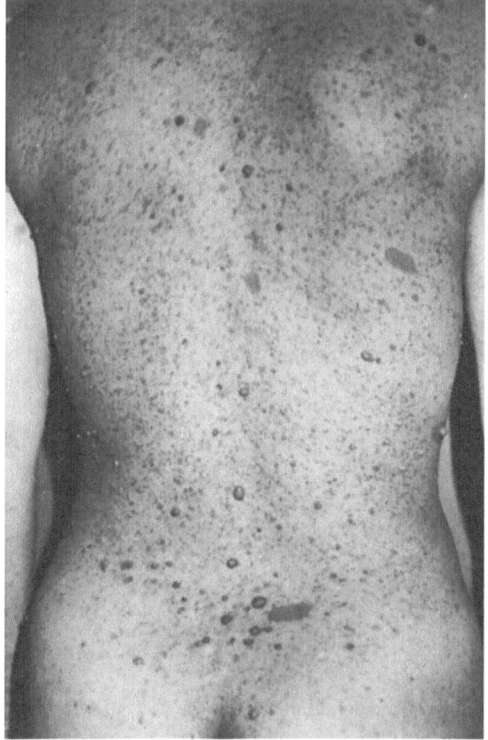

Fig. 14.6. Neurofibromatosis: gross cutaneous lesions.

Neurofibromata occur on peripheral nerves and can involve cranial nerves (acoustic neuroma) or nerves emerging from the spinal cord, giving rise to cord or root compression. Mental retardation is not uncommon and hypertension due to associated phaeochromocytoma is an occasional complication. A small percentage of tumours undergo sarcomatous change.

Up to 50% of affected children have scoliosis with a rapidly progressive, short, sharp curve, involving four or five vertebrae.

Fibrous replacement or interosseous cystic lesions may occur in bones and lead to fracture and pseudarthrosis. The classical and commonest site is in the lower tibia, but the lesions have also been encountered in the fibula, ulna and clavicle (Richin et al. 1976; Brown et al. 1977). Hypertrophy of a single bone, digit or an entire limb may develop. The presence of more than five smoothly outlined pigmented macules, which are more than 1.5 cm in diameter, is generally accepted as being diagnostic of neurofibromatosis. However, these criteria are by no means absolute and a diagnostic dilemma often arises when children with a few lesions of this type present with a kyphoscoliosis.

Radiographic Appearances

There are no pathognomic radiographic appearances. Local hypertrophy of a bone or a limb may be present, but in these circumstances the bones are of normal shape. A short-curve kyphoscoliosis may be apparent in early childhood and although cysts or

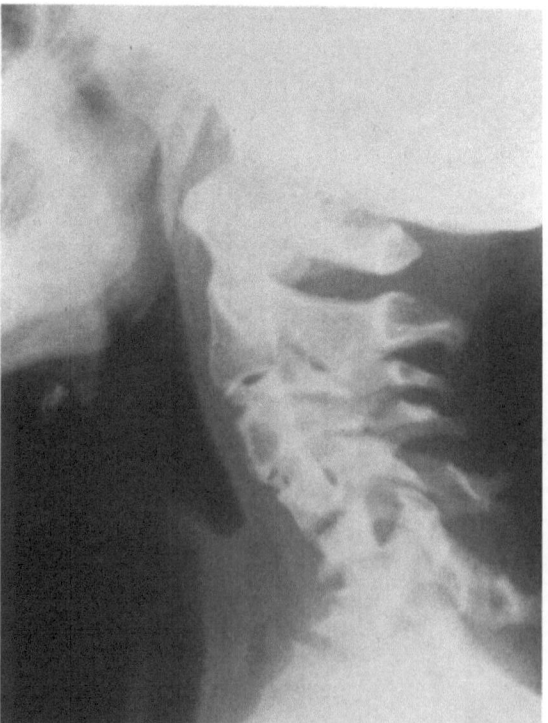

Fig. 14.7. Neurofibromatosis: radiograph of cervical spine of an adolescent girl, showing severe deformity. Courtesy of Mr. D. H. Jones, Bangor.

areas of fibrous replacement of bone have been seen at birth (Sprague and Brown 1974) these more commonly become manifest a little later (Fig. 14.7). Radiographs of established tibial pseudarthrosis show complete fracture with bowing, which is proximal or distal to the fracture site, sclerotic tapering bone ends, absence of callus and loss of medullary space. Lesions which are situated within intervertebral foramina may cause local bone erosion (Fig. 14.8). The radiographic changes have been reviewed by Holt and Wright (1948) and Hunt and Pugh (1961).

Genetics

Neurofibromatosis is inherited as an autosomal dominant with very variable clinical expression.

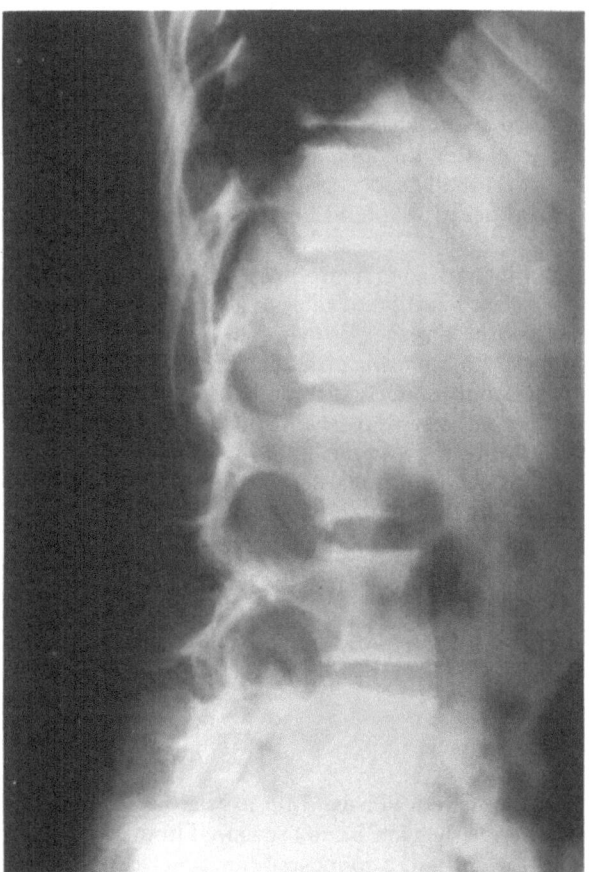

Fig. 14.8. Neurofibromatosis: lateral radiograph of the thoraco-lumbar spine showing marked enlargement of the nerve root foramina.

Management

The scoliosis is rapidly progressive and as it is not controllable by a Milwaukee brace, early operative stabilisation and fusion are required.

The management of pseudarthrosis of the tibia is an orthopaedic nightmare and a continual trial to those dealing with the problem. Typically, the fracture occurs in the first 2 years of life and is usually preceeded by anterior and medial bowing of the tibia. After fracture union is rarely achieved without operation (Nichol 1969). Various procedures have been advocated which fall into three broad categories: Nichol (1969) excised the abnormal area and used a double onlay corticocancellous graft, McFarland (1951), Eyre-Brook et al. (1969) and Lloyd-Roberts and Shaw (1969) advised bypass grafting and others (Charnley 1956; Van Ness 1966) have advocated intramedullary nailing. If union can be achieved, protection by a polythene gaiter is required until the late teens since refracture is possible. However, after the age of eight union seems to be achieved much more readily (Lloyd-Roberts 1971). Recently promising results have been obtained where other methods have failed by the use of prolonged exposure to pulsed electromagnetic fields (Sutcliffe et al. 1979) or direct current stimulation (Paterson et al. 1980).

Richin et al. (1976) described the management of a boy who had an established pseudarthrosis of the junction of the middle and lower third of the radius and ulna which was evident at birth. Delivery was by Caesarian section and there was no suggestion of perinatal trauma. The lesion was managed by distraction splinting. No attempt had been made to gain union by the time the child was 5 years of age, since the lesion was free of pain and there was good function with no requirement for bearing weight. Manske (1979) described a similar lesion which was sustained at the age of three. This fracture failed to join after immobilisation in plaster and later internal fixation. Internal fixation was eventually successful in attaining union at the age of 13, and the author suggested that operation should be delayed until this age in such patients.

Although there have been reports of intraosseous neurofibromata and schwannomas, neurofibromatous tissue has not been identified at the site of a non-union, even when there has been clinical evidence of the disease. Brown et al. (1977) examined specimens from the site of non-union in 17 patients with pseudarthrosis of the tibia of whom eight had clinical evidence of neurofibromatosis, three had fibrous dysplasia and six had no evidence of either. The sections were examined by both light and electron microscopy but were histologically indistinguishable.

Lesions which give rise to root or cord compression will require early decompression and removal of the neurofibroma if this is possible (Curtis et al. 1969).

Neurofibromata may enlarge during pregnancy and in these circumstances paraplegia may be the consequence of swelling of a lesion in the spinal canal.

14.4 Fibrous Dysplasia

The fibrous dysplasias do not have a genetic basis, but as they share some characteristics with the preceding conditions they are briefly reviewed in this section.

Two forms of fibrous dysplasia are recognised, a monostotic in which lesions are confined to a single bone and a polyostotic in which bone changes are widespread. In this latter type areas of irregular cutaneous café-au-lait pigmentation may be present, and in approximately 3% of these patients endocrine changes promote premature sexual development, when the condition is termed the 'McCune-Albright syndrome'.

Clinical Features

The monostotic form is the most common and the lesions may be asymptomatic and recognised only on an incidental radiograph. The most common sites are the proximal femur, the tibia, the ribs and the face; the presenting features are pain, fracture or bony swelling, usually in the second or third decade of life. Cutaneous pigmentation is said to be rare in the monostotic variety. The skeletal lesions may be static or gradually fill and expand the bone, producing deformity. Progress is uncommon after puberty.

Changes may be widespread in the polyostotic form. Harris et al. (1962) found that 25% of their patients had more than half the skeleton involved and the majority of these experienced symptoms before the age of ten. The lesion may have segmental distribution in a single extremity. If severe skeletal problems appear early, multiple fractures and deformities may be anticipated. The cranio-facial structures are affected in about half the patients with the polyostotic form, but spinal changes are uncommon. Albright's syndrome is almost entirely restricted to girls. These children have precocious sexual development, rapid bone maturation, and early epiphyseal closure with consequent short stature.

The cutaneous lesions are multiple, well-demarcated, flat melanotic areas which stop at the mid-line and have irregular margins. This configuration has been likened to the indented 'coast of Maine' in distinction to the smooth 'coast of California' outline of the pigmented macules in neurofibromatosis.

Radiographic Appearances

Typically there is a large radiolucent area in a long bone, and if the fibrous tissue contains sufficient osseous material a 'ground glass' appearance may result (Fig. 14.9). The changes may involve a segment or the entire bone. The periosteum is not breached unless there is a fracture but lesions near the periphery of a long bone may produce erosion and scalloping of the cortex. The upper femur often presents a characteristic 'shepherd's crook' deformity. Fracture healing is normal, with periosteal callus formation. Patients with severe facial involvement may show localised bony hyperplasia.

Management

The orthopaedic management of fibrous dysplasia has been well summarised by Grabias and Campbell (1977). No medical treatment is available to prevent progression of the lesions in polyostotic disease. Radiotherapy is valueless and may induce malignant change. Monostotic lesions are operated upon for biopsy and diagnosis, and to eliminate the defect by curettage and grafting, for which any suitable bone may be used. Many single lesions have been observed to slowly reossify if left alone. Fractures should be treated conventionally in children, with emphasis on functional bracing. Fractures involving severe femoral or tibial deformity will require open reduction and internal fixation. The femoral shepherd's crook deformity may be treated by multiple osteotomies and fixation with a Zickel nail or a Küntscher nail and signal arm (Y nail) attachment. Intramedullary fixation is preferable to plates and screws.

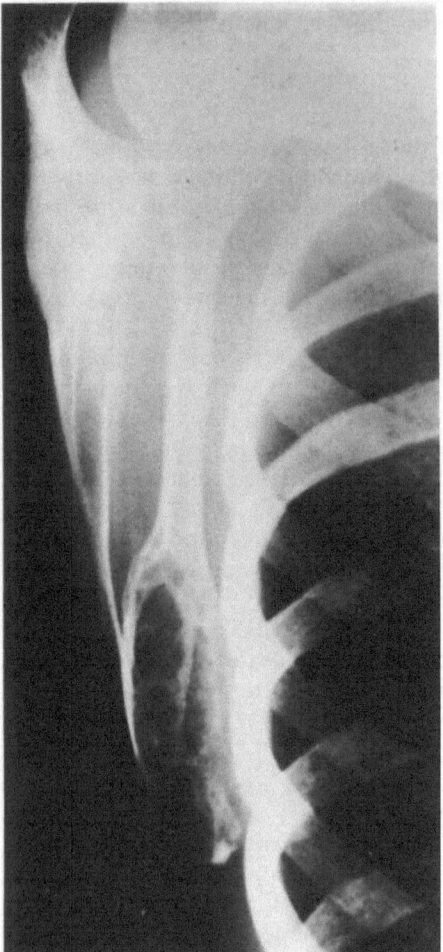

Fig. 14.9. Fibrous dysplasia of the scapula.

Malignant change occurs in about 1% of the lesions. The most common form of malignancy is osteosarcoma, but because of the multiple constituents of the abnormal fibrous tissue, chondrosarcoma, fibrosarcoma and giant cell tumours may arise; a rhabdomyosarcoma has recently been reported (Johnson et al. 1979).

14.5 Fibrodysplasia Ossificans Progressiva (F.O.P.)

This uncommon genetic disease is also known as myositis ossificans progressiva, but the designation 'fibrodysplasia ossificans progressiva' is to be preferred as it is a more accurate reflection of the underlying pathological process.

Clinical Features

A short hallux (Fig. 14.10) and sometimes a short thumb may be present at birth but the characteristic inflamed swellings appear at any time from infancy to adulthood. These most commonly develop in late childhood and the sites of predilection are the upper back, neck and shoulders (Figs. 14.11 and 14.12). The lesions subside over a week or two but eventually they calcify and ossify. Initially there may be no more than mild trunk stiffness but as the disease progresses the fascial planes, tendon attachments and intermuscular septa ossify. The bony plaques gradually become widespread and the patient may eventually become completely immobile.

The progression of the disease is variable, but the general health often remains surprisingly unimpaired despite considerable restriction of movement. Respiratory failure may eventually supervene, but those patients with less extensive ossification may live until old age. Shortening of the thumbs and great toes is an important diagnostic pointer and permits differentiation from other disorders in which widespread tissue calcification is prominent.

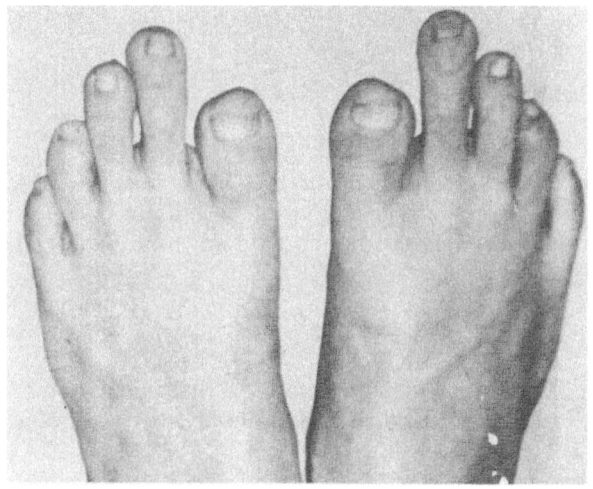

▲
Fig. 14.10. Fibrodysplasia ossificans progressiva: short hallux.

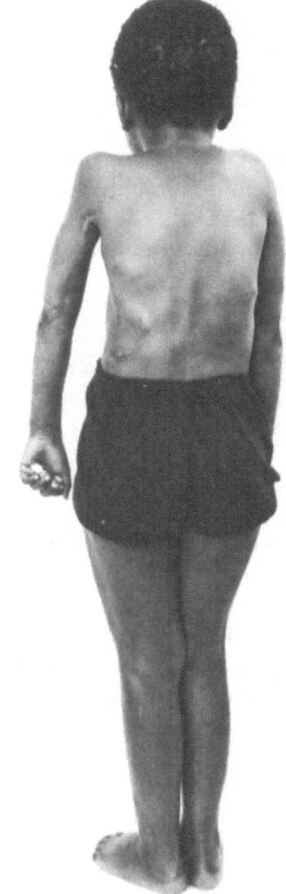

Fig. 14.11. Fibrodysplasia ossificans progressiva: typical lesions on back and shoulders. ▶

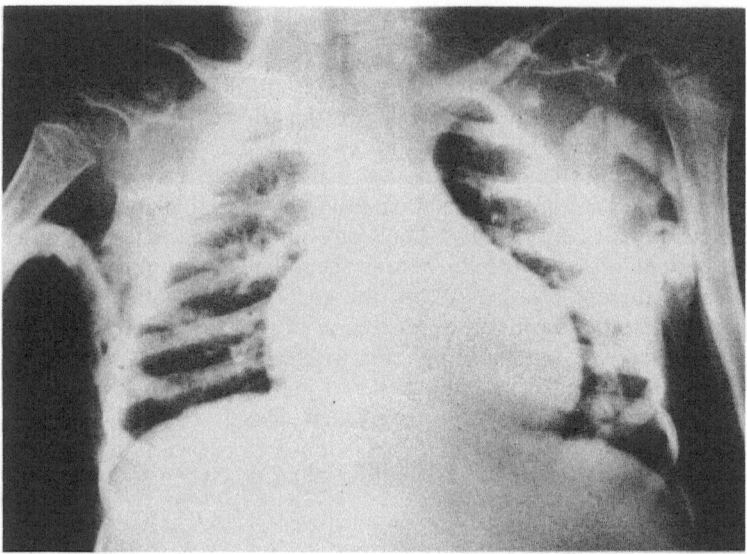

Fig. 14.12. Fibrodysplasia ossificans progressiva: radiograph showing calcified plaques across back and axillae.

Radiographic Appearances

Radiographs show shortening and maldevelopment of the first metatarsal and the phalanges of the associated first ray. Plaques of bone are visible usually in line with muscle planes or at tendon attachments. Bone struts may be laid down in the fascial planes across joints, abolishing mobility.

Genetics

Fibrodysplasia ossificans progressiva is inherited as an autosomal dominant, but as severely affected patients rarely reproduce the majority are probably the result of a new mutation.

Management

The aims of treatment are to prevent the formation of ectopic bone which causes fixation of joints and progressive immobility, and to increase mobility in patients who are already crippled (Smith et al. 1976). There is evidence to suggest that steroids may help to suppress the acute inflammatory process (Eaton et al. 1957; Illingworth 1971) but this form of therapy does not appear to inhibit calcification. Joint stiffness is partly due to the formation of fibrous tissue and the matrix in which calcification will ultimately occur, and therefore attempts at decalcifying established plaques or delaying ossification will have a limited value. Dietary restriction of calcium or Vitamin D does not reduce heterotopic mineralisation.

The diphosphonate EHDP prevents the formation and dissolution of apatite crystals in vitro and has been shown to suppress osteoblastic activity in Paget disease (Russell et al. 1974). It has been used in F.O.P. to prevent mineralisation of areas of active myositis or recurrence after removal of established areas of calcification, with variable success (Smith et al. 1976). These workers also consider that EHDP is not effective when bone is removed in the active phase of the disease, but that it may help to suppress recalcification after operation in the inactive stage. Uncertainty as to the amount of EHDP which is actually absorbed makes estimation of an optimum schedule of dosage difficult.

Surgical removal of established plaques of bone is of some value in attempting to improve movements in the severely crippled, but the incidence of reformation is extremely high. Surgical adjustment of the stiff limbs to a position of optimum function is perhaps the most valuable procedure that can be offered to the profoundly disabled patient. By this means a degree of self-care may be retained in terms of the requirements of feeding and personal hygiene.

References

Diaphyseal Aclasia

Barnes R, Catto M (1966) Chondrosarcoma of bone. J Bone Joint Surg [Br] 48:729
Clark LP, Atwood CE (1907) A case of multiple enchondroma, one of which is growing from the sella turcica causing pressure on the pituitary body, the chiasm and crura. NY State J. Med 86:102
Epstein DA, Levin EJ (1978) Bone scintigraphy in hereditary multiple exostoses. Am J Roentgenol 130:331
Keith A (1919) Studies on the anatomical changes which accompany certain growth disorders of the human body. Anat 54:101
Roman G (1978) Hereditary multiple exostoses. A rare cause of spinal cord compression. Spine 3:230
Weiner DS, Hoyt WA Jr. (1978) Clin Orthop 137:187

Enchondromatosis

Elmore SM, Cantrill WC (1966) Maffucci's syndrome. A case report with a normal karyotype. J. Bone Joint Surg [Am] 48:1607
Giannikas AC (1966) Treatment of metacarpal enchondromata. Report of three cases. J Bone Joint Surg [Br] 48:333
Lewis RJ, Ketcham AS (1973) Maffucci's syndrome: functional neoplastic significance. Case report and a review of the literature. J Bone Joint Surg [Am] 55:1965
Maffucci A (1881) Di un caso di enchondroma ed angioma multiple. Morgagni 3:399
Mosher JF (1976) Multiple enchondromatosis of the hand. A case report. J Bone Joint Surg [Am] 58:717
Takigawa K (1971) Chondroma of the bones of the hand. A review of 110 cases. J Bone Joint Surg [Am] 53:1951

Neurofibromatosis

Brown GA, Osebold WR, Ponsetti IV (1977) Congenital pseudarthrosis of long bones. Clin Orthop 128:228
Charnley J (1956) Congenital pseudarthrosis of the tibia treated by the intramedullary nail. J Bone Joint Surg [Am] 38:283
Curtis BM, Fisher RL, Butterfield WL, Saunders FP (1969) Neurofibromatosis with paraplegia. Report of 8 cases. J Bone Joint Surg [Am] 51:843
Eyre-Brook AL, Baily AJ, Price CHG (1969) Infantile pseudoarthrosis of the tibia. J Bone Joint Surg [Br] 51:604
Holt JF, Wright EM (1948) The radiological features of neurofibromatosis. Radiology 51:647
Hunt JC, Puch DG (1961) Skeletal lesions in neurofibromatosis. Radiology 76:1

Lloyd-Roberts GC, Shaw NE (1969) The prevention of pseudoarthrosis in congenital kyphosis of the tibia. J Bone Joint Surg [Br] 51:100

McFarland B (1951) Pseudoarthrosis of the tibia in childhood. J Bone Joint Surg [Br] 33:36

Manske PR (1979) Forearm pseudoarthrosis-neurofibromatosis. A case report. Clin Orthop 139:125

Nicoll EA (1969) Infantile pseudoarthrosis of the tibia. J Bone Joint Surg [Br] 51:589

Paterson DC, Lewis GN, Cass CA (1980) Treatment of congenital pseudoarthrosis of the tibia with direct current stimulation. Clin Orthop 148:129

Richin PF Kranik A, Van Herpe L, Suffecool SL (1976) Congenital pseudoarthrosis of both bones of the forearm. A case report. J Bone Joint Surg [Am] 58:1032

Sprague BL, Brown GA (1974) Congenital pseudoarthrosis of the radius. J Bone Joint Surg [Am] 56:191

Sutcliffe ML, Sharrard WJW, MacEachern G (1980) The treatment of fracture union by electromagnetic induction. J Bone Joint Surg [Br] 62:123

Van Ness CP (1966) Congenital pseudoarthrosis of the leg. J Bone Joint Surg [Am] 48:1467

Wellwood JM, Bulmer JH, Graff DJC (1971) Congenital defects of the tibia in siblings with neurofibromatosis. J Bone Joint Surg [Br] 53:314

Fibrous Dysplasia

Grabias SL, Campbell CJ (1977) Fibrous dysplasia. Clin Orthop 8:771

Harris W, Dudley R, Barry R (1962) The natural history of fibrous dysplasia. J Bone Joint Surg [Am] 44:207

Johnson CB, Gilbert EF, Gottlieb LI (1979) Malignant transformation of polyostotic fibrous dysplasia. South Med 72:353

Fibrodysplasia Ossificans Progressiva

Eaton WL, Conkling WS, Daeschner CW (1957) Early myositis ossificans progressiva occurring in homozygotic twins. A clinical and pathological study. J Pediatr 50:591

Illingworth RS (1971) Myositis ossificans progressiva (Munchmeyer's disease) Brief review with report of two cases treated with corticosteroids and observed for 16 years. Arch Dis Child 46:264

Russell RGG, Smith R, Preston S, Walton RJ, Woods C (1974) Diphosphonates in Paget's disease. Lancet 1:894

Smith R, Russell RGG, Woods CG (1976) Myositis ossificans progressiva. J Bone Joint Surg [Br] 58:48

15. Miscellaneous Disorders

The difficulties of classifying the bone dysplasias in a satisfactory manner have been discussed in Chapter 3, where the reasons for adopting the arrangement which has been used in this book were explained. It is inevitable that a number of disorders fail to fit into a convenient category and these have been reviewed in this chapter.

15.1 Osteopoikilosis

Osteopoikilosis is usually diagnosed by chance following radiography for an unrelated purpose, when the characteristic appearance of 'spotty bones' is recognised.

Clinical Features

There are usually no clinical manifestations although some patients are said to have had unexplained joint pains, and about 15% have patches of multiple sessile dermal nodules known as 'dermatofibrosis lenticularis disseminata'.

Radiographic Appearances

Numerous sclerotic symmetrical bone islands between 3 and 5 mm in diameter are seen (Fig. 15.1), principally at the ends of the long bones. In children they are present in the epiphyses as well as the metaphyses. There is no other bony abnormality.

Genetics

Osteopoikilosis is inherited as an autosomal dominant trait.

Management

Osteopoikilosis is generally regarded as an interesting condition of no clinical significance. However, Mindell et al. (1978) have reported a man aged 48 with osteopoikilosis, who developed an osteosarcoma at the upper end of his left tibia. The lesion was subjected to intensive histological assessment and osteoblastic activity was observed in a bone island immediately adjacent to the osteosarcoma. These authors suggested that there may be a relationship between the two conditions.

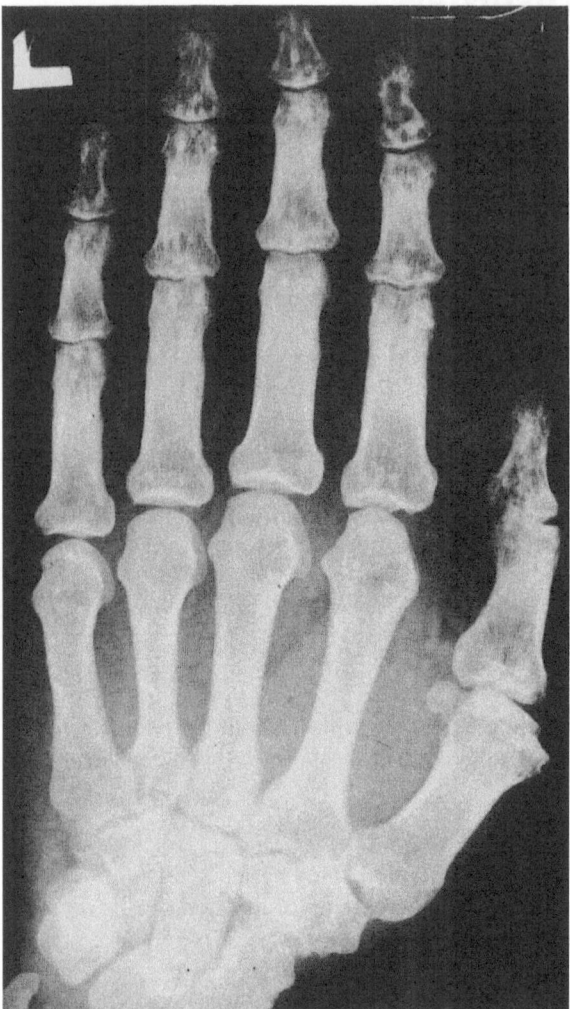

Fig. 15.1. Osteopoikilosis.

15.2 Melorheostosis

Melorheostosis is a rare non-genetic condition in which soft tissue contractures and skin abnormalities are associated with linear hyperostosis of the long bones. The name, which is derived from the Greek, pertains to the characteristic radiological appearance of the hyperostosis, which resembles wax running down the cortex of the bone.

Clinical Features

Melorheostosis is usually monomelic and may be monostotic or polyostotic. The limb girdles may be involved but the skull, spine and ribs are usually spared. The affected extremity may commonly be shorter but is occasionally longer than its normal fellow.

In children pain is infrequent and never severe and the principal problems are soft tissue contracture and limb inequality (Young et al. 1979). Joint contractures may be present at an early age and there is sometimes delay in reaching the true diagnosis due to confusion with arthrogryposis. The contractures are often severe and resistant to treatment.

Affected adults may be asymptomatic but the majority of patients complain of pain, which is usually related to the region of the bone lesion. This pain varies in quality from dull to sharp, is rarely severe or constant and worsens after activity. There is usually associated joint stiffness which may be the result of soft tissue contracture, fibrosis or involvement of the joint surface by hyperostosis. The skin overlying the bone lesion is often shiny and erythematous.

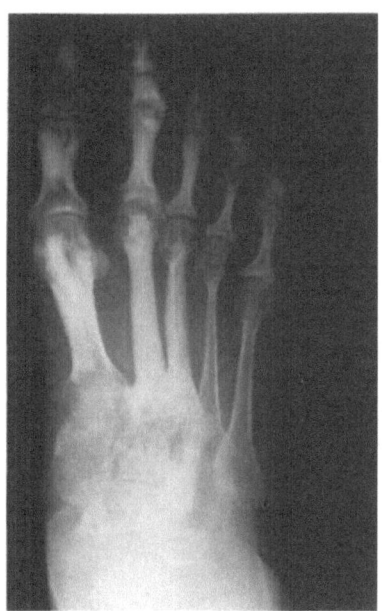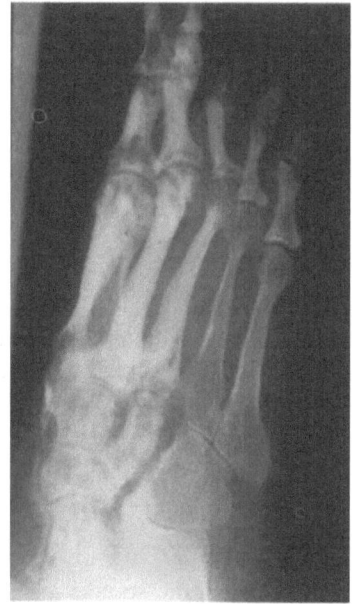

Fig. 15.2. Melorheostosis.

Radiographic Appearances (Fig. 15.2)

There is an irregular, linear hyperostosis along the cortices of long bones, with a distinct demarcation between normal and abnormal. The hyperostosis may extend down the limb from one bone to the next and 'flow' into the tarsus or carpus. In the early stages of the disease the joints are spared, but in well established cases they may be invaded by hyperostotic bone.

The flat bones tend to have patches and streaks of sclerosis and the epiphyseal areas may have a spotted appearance. In children the radiographic changes differ in that the hyperostosis appears to be endosteal without the 'flowing' cortical thickening. Streaking of long bones and spotting of the tarsus, carpus and epiphyses may be seen in these patients.

Management

The management of melorheostosis in children has been reviewed by Young et al. (1979) and in children and adults by Campbell et al. (1968).

The soft tissue contractures in children are extremely resistant to treatment and although correction may be obtained at operation relapse almost invariably occurs. Distal ischaemia may be encountered when correcting severe soft tissue contractures of the knee, and supracondylar femoral osteotomy is preferable to soft tissue release to shorten as well as straighten the limb.

Contractures tend to progress less slowly in adults but correction is equally disappointing with a high rate of relapse. In extreme circumstances amputation may be required for persistent pain and deformity.

15.3 Osteopathia Striata

Voorhoeve initially described the appearances of multiple linear sclerotic streaking on radiographs of the long bones and pelvis in 1924. The term osteopathia striata was applied to the condition by Sir Thomas Fairbank in 1935.

Clinical Features

There are no clinical features and the diagnosis is made solely on radiographic examination. Similar striations are sometimes seen in association with osteopetrosis, osteopoikilosis and focal dermal hypoplasia (Goltz syndrome). Osteopathia striata with basal skull thickening, mild facial distortion and cranial nerve palsies is a distinct familial disorder which is inherited as an autosomal dominant (Walker 1969; Horan and Beighton 1978).

Radiographic Appearances

Multiple parallel linear hyperostotic streaks are seen in the metaphyses of the long bones (Fig. 15.3). The streaking is also characteristically present in the iliac bones where it has a fan-like distribution.

Genetics

Voorhoeve's original paper concerned a father and a daughter, and autosomal dominant inheritance is well established.

Management

Isolated osteopathia striata requires no treatment but when basal skull sclerosis is also present, decompression of the 7th and 8th cranial nerves may be necessary.

Major limb defects are a complication of focal dermal hypoplasia. These are very variable in terms of anatomical involvement, but merit orthopaedic management in their own right.

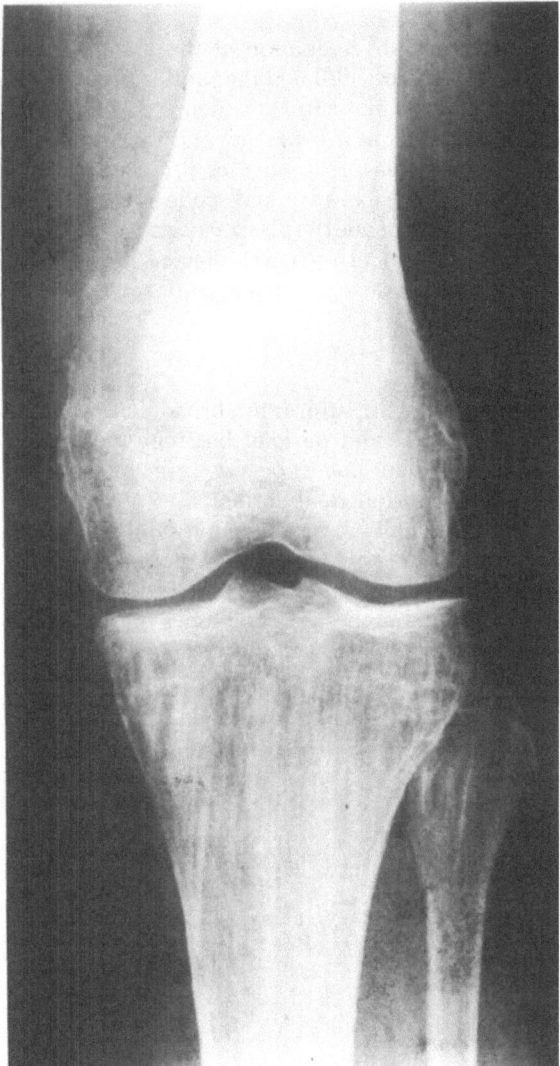

Fig. 15.3. Osteopathia striata.

15.4 Cleidocranial Dysplasia

Cleidocranial dysplasia was first recognised by Martin in 1765 and the syndrome was delineated and termed 'cranio-cleidal dysostosis' by Marie and Sainton in 1897. Initially the abnormalities were thought to be restricted to the skull and clavicle, but the realisation that a widespread skeletal maldevelopment was frequently present led to the adoption of the term 'dysplasia' rather than 'dysostosis' at the Paris nomenclature meeting in 1969.

Clinical Features

The syndrome is sometimes recognised at birth by palpation of the incompletely ossified calvarium (Fauré and Maroteaux 1973). In childhood the skull is broad with frontal and parietal bossing and closure of the cranial sutures is delayed. The teeth may be poorly aligned, small and deformed. The chest is narrow and the shoulders are unusually mobile anteriorly due to hypoplasia or absence of the clavicles.

Orthopaedic complications are uncommon but coxa vara and scoliosis sometimes develop and may require treatment. Occasionally pelvic dysplasia causes problems at childbirth and Caesarian section may be necessary. In general affected individuals have few problems and they are usually able to lead a normal and active life.

Radiographic Appearances

In the newborn the skull is undermineralised and the sutures are broad. The skull is slow to ossify and is brachycephalic with frontal and parietal bossing. Closure of sutures and fontanelles is delayed and wormian bones persist (Fig. 15.4). The mid-facial skeleton is underdeveloped and dentition is abnormal.

The clavicles are sometimes absent but are usually represented by small medial or lateral stumps (Fig. 15.5). The scapulae are dysplastic and minor anomalies of the bones of the hands and feet are common. The thorax is usually narrowed and shows delayed maturation of the vertebrae; vertebral anomalies are sometimes present. The pelvic bones are slow to ossify and may be hypoplastic at maturity (Fig. 15.6). The femoral necks are occasionally deformed and bilateral coxa vara may develop.

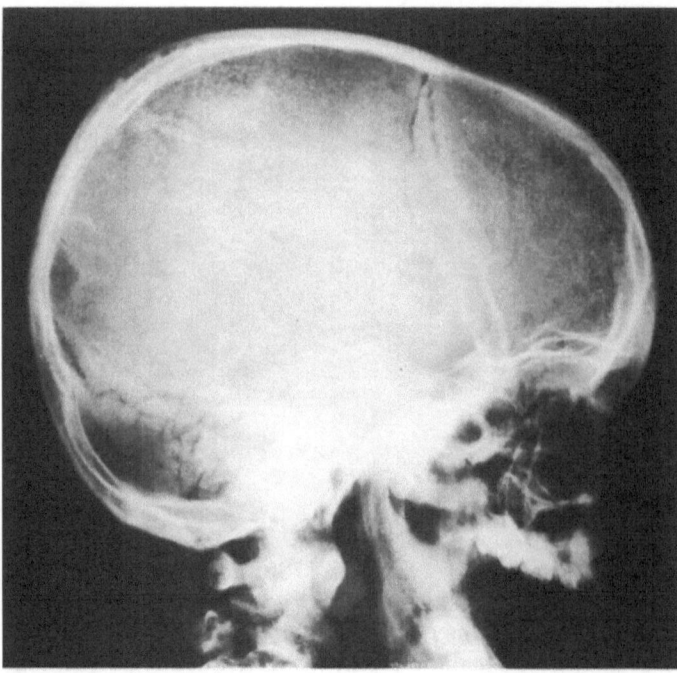

Fig. 15.4. Cleidocranial dysplasia. Lateral view of adolescent skull showing delayed closure of the cranial sutures, wormian bones and mid-facial hypoplasia.

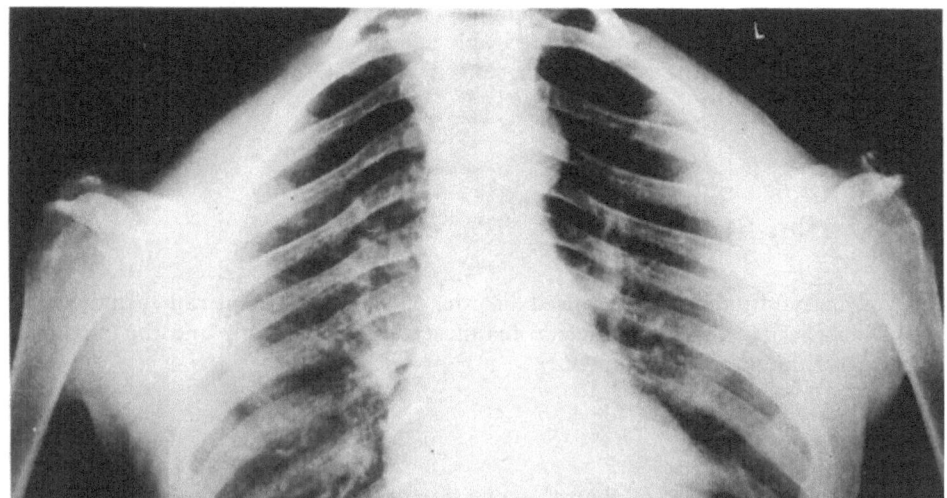

Fig. 15.5. Cleidocranial dysplasia. The clavicles are represented by small lateral remnants.

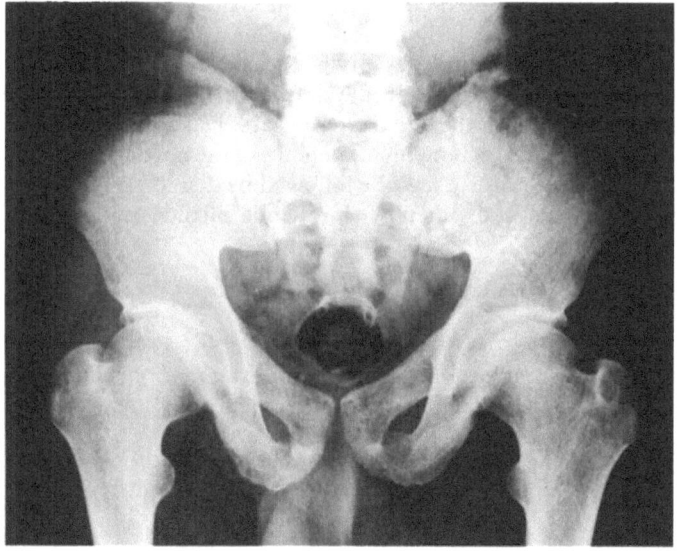

Fig. 15.6. Cleidocranial dysplasia. Mild pelvic hypoplasia, short femoral necks.

Genetics

Cleidocranial dysplasia is inherited as an autosomal dominant trait with variable clinical expression.

Management

Abnormal teeth frequently necessitate dental attention. The incidence of coxa vara is uncertain but when present it should be managed in the standard manner by valgus osteotomy of the upper end of the femur. The hypoplastic clavicles present few problems and intervention is neither desirable nor required, although there is a single report of brachial plexus compression caused by a lateral clavicular stump.

15.5 Marfan Syndrome

The Marfan syndrome is a generalised disorder of connective tissue rather than a true bone dysplasia. However, the skeletal manifestations are striking and the condition merits description in this chapter.

Clinical Features (Fig. 15.7)

There is a wide spectrum of clinical expression and many patients are only mildly affected. The length of the limbs is increased in relation to the trunk, with the lower segment (pubis to heel) measurement exceeding the upper (crown to pubis). Similarly the arm span is greater than the height. The digits are disproportionately long and slim (arachnodactyly) and some patients have joint laxity which may result in persistent dislocation of the patella and shoulder. The feet are usually flat and hypermobile, hallux valgus is often seen and pes cavus occasionally occurs.

About 50% of patients with the Marfan syndrome develop a moderate to severe scoliosis which may progress rapidly from the age of 9–10 years. Pectus excavatum is often present. Cardiovascular problems include incompetence of the aortic and mitral valves while aneurysm formation in the aorta may be followed by dissection. Bilateral ectopia lentis is a consistent feature and other eye problems include myopia and retinal detachment.

Radiographic Appearances

There are no pathognomonic appearances on radiographic examination. However, the unusual length of the tubular bones of the hands and feet is readily apparent and there may be a scoliosis without obvious bony deformity.

Genetics

The Marfan syndrome is inherited as an autosomal dominant trait with variable expression.

Management

Many patients are not severely affected and require no active treatment. In young girls hormones have been administered in order to inhibit growth and thus prevent extreme height and minimise the risk of scoliosis.

A scoliosis which warrants treatment will need initial management with a Milwaukee brace, but if this fails reduction and fusion using Harrington rods is required (Robins et al. 1974). Progression may be rapid and careful monitoring of the early curve is necessary.

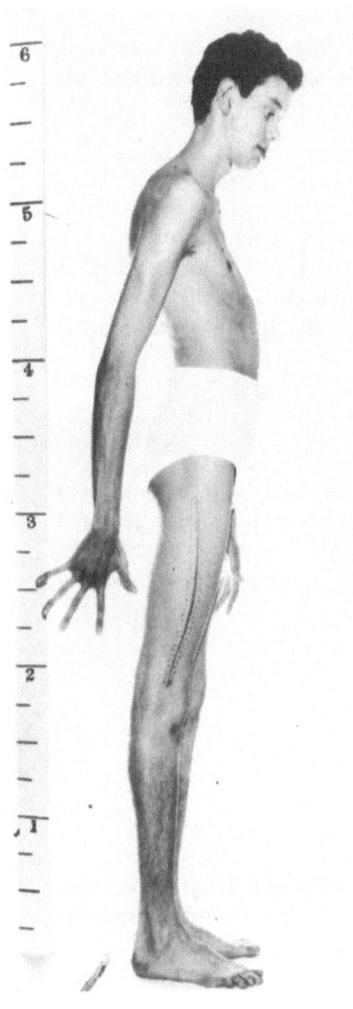

Fig. 15.7. The Marfan syndrome: increased limb length, arachnodactyly, pes planus and mild pectus excavatus in an adolescent.

Foot problems present difficulties with shoe fitting and operative correction of hallux valgus and hammer toe may be required. Occasionally subtalar fusion is necessary for painful planovalgus feet.

In view of the high frequency of abnormalities of the heart, the cardiovascular state should be carefully assessed before anaesthesia and operation.

15.6 Homocystinuria

Homocystinuria and the Marfan syndrome have many common features and at the clinical level diagnostic confusion sometimes arises. However, they differ in their pathogenesis, as homocystinuria is an autosomal recessively inherited inborn error of methionine metabolism, whereas the Marfan syndrome is an autosomal dominant connective tissue disorder.

Clinical Features

The principal clinical characteristics of the established disease are a Marfanoid habitus with ectopia lentis and progressive mental retardation, with or without fits. Thromboembolism is a frequent complication.

Radiographic Appearances

The changes, which are age-related, have been reviewed by Thomas and Carson (1977). Vertebral flattening and anterior wedging giving rise to kyphosis which is present in some degree in all but the most mildly affected patients. In the long bones there is marked increase in length in late childhood, with large epiphyses and broad metaphyses.

Management

There are two types of homocystinuria, one of which responds to treatment with pyridoxine whilst the other is pyridoxine resistant and requires a diet which is low in methionine. The tendency to thromboembolism is a major surgical hazard and operation should be avoided if possible. Consequently the management of skeletal problems is essentially conservative.

15.7 Larsen Syndrome

The Larsen syndrome is probably not uncommon and although joint laxity pre-dominates over the primary skeletal changes the condition warrants consideration by virtue of the potentially serious orthopaedic complications.

Clinical Features

Children with the Larsen syndrome present at birth as 'floppy babies' and their generalised joint laxity may be associated with dislocation of the hips or radial heads, dislocation or subluxation of the knees and talipes equinovarus. The mid-portion of the face is underdeveloped giving a 'dish' appearance and there is flattening of the bridge of the nose (Figs. 15.8 and 15.9). The terminal phalanges of the digits have a spatulate configuration and the thumbs are broad. Stature is short and in some patients this problem is compounded by a severe kyphoscoliosis. Structural cardiac defects may be present in the recessive form of the disorder.

Radiographic Appearances

Multiple joint dislocations may be seen at the hips, knees and elbows and hemivertebrae and spinal malalignment are often present. The calcaneum has an extra ossification centre which appears in late infancy and supernumary ossicles are evident in the carpus.

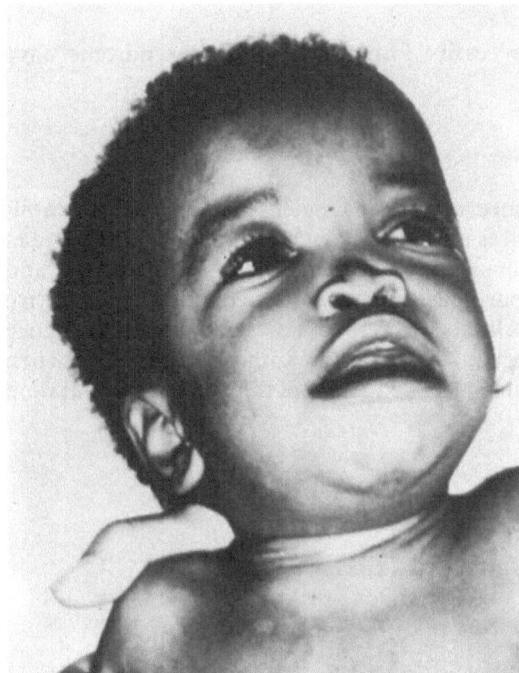

Fig. 15.8. Larsen syndrome: mid-facial hypoplasia and flattening of the nasal bridge give a 'dish' appearance.

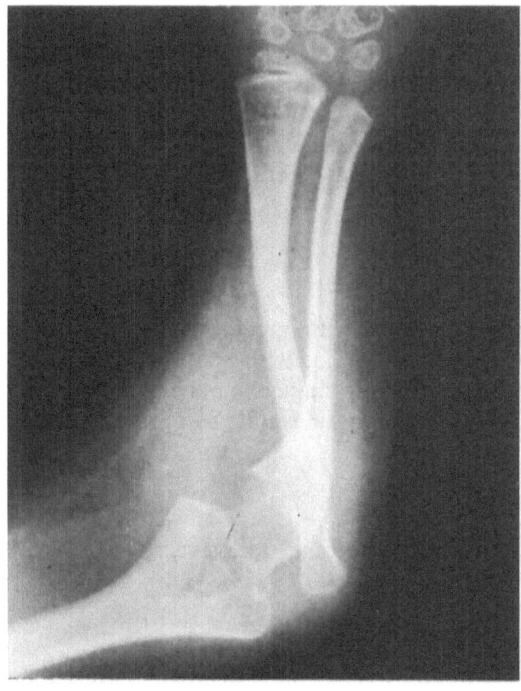

Fig. 15.9. Larsen syndrome: dislocation of radial head and elbow.

Genetics

Autosomal dominant and autosomal recessive forms of the Larsen syndrome have been reported.

Management

The principal orthopaedic problems concern the management of major joint instability and dislocations, especially of the knees and hips. Larsen et al. (1950) and Latta et al. (1971) found that attempts at conservative treatment by manipulation and maintenance of reduction in plaster of paris casts invariably failed, and that operative reduction was necessary. However, Oki et al. (1976) successfully treated knee dislocation by traction shortly after birth. These latter authors stated that when closed reduction of the knee had been achieved, reduction of the hip by manipulation was then possible.

15.8 Chondro-Ectodermal Dysplasia (Ellis-Van Creveld Syndrome)

This uncommon disorder has been studied principally among the Amish, an inbred religious isolate in Pennsylvania, although it has occasionally been observed in other population groups.

Clinical Features

Disproportionate dwarfism with shortening of the limbs which is more marked in the middle and distal portions (acromesomelia) is the major feature. Post-axial polydactyly is often present in the hands but is much less common in the feet. The nails are hypoplastic, the hair is fine and sparse and the teeth are abnormal. The upper lip may be partially fused to the mucosa of the upper jaw. Structural cardiac defects occur in about 50% of the patients.

Radiographic Appearances

The tubular bones show progressive distal shortening with hypoplasia of the terminal phalanges. The pelvis is underdeveloped in early childhood with small iliac wings and acetabular deformity, but these appearances gradually change to normal in later life. Dysplasia of the lateral part of the upper tibial epiphysis results in genu valgum.

Genetics

Chondro-ectodermal dysplasia is inherited as an autosomal recessive.

Management

The cardiac complications can be lethal in infancy. Removal of the extra digit will be required if it is interfering with hand function. The genu valgum may necessitate varus osteotomy but the deformity may recur before skeletal growth is completed and repeated operative correction may be required.

15.9 Schwartz Syndrome

The Schwartz syndrome is a rare disorder in which skeletal dysplasia, short stature and myotonia predispose to a variety of orthopaedic complications.

Clinical Features

There is a mask-like facies with blepharophimosis and ptosis. Progressive contractures of the hips, knees and elbows occur and talipes equinovarus is a consistent finding. All the joints are stiff and the gait is a mere shuffle. The myotonia is progressive until it reaches a plateau in mid-childhood. The long bones of the limbs may become bowed and kyphoscoliosis sometimes develops (Fig. 15.10).

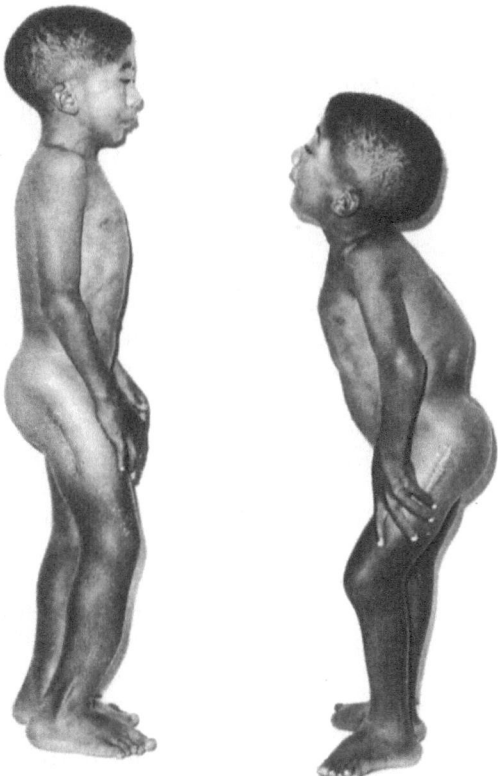

Fig. 15.10. The Schwartz syndrome in two brothers.

Radiographic Appearances

The skeleton is undermineralised. Moderate platyspondyly is present and wedging of the vertebral bodies may cause kyphosis. The epiphyses and metaphyses are dysplastic and the knees may show varus or valgus deformities. The hips may be dislocated and coxa vara and valga have been reported.

Genetics

The Schwartz syndrome is inherited as an autosomal recessive.

Management

Operation for talipes equinovarus and congenital hip dislocation has been successful and correction of fixed flexion at the knees by supracondylar osteotomy of the femur has also been carried out. Problems with the induction of anaesthesia may arise because of the small mouth, rigidity of the temporomandibular joint, myotonia and the short stiff neck (Horan and Beighton 1975).

15.10 Dyschondrosteosis

Dyschondrosteosis is characterised by moderate short stature due to shortening of the forearm and lower leg (mesomelia) and a Madelung deformity of the wrist. The restricted growth and wrist abnormality become apparent in mid-childhood, but there are no other notable problems. Inheritance is autosomal dominant with more marked expression in females.

15.10.1 The Madelung Deformity

In 1878 Madelung described volar subluxation of the carpus on the radius, which he attributed to a disturbance in growth of the distal radial epiphyses. In the established deformity the radius is short and curved; there is dorsal subluxation of the distal end of the ulna and mild volar subluxation of the radiocarpal joint with restriction of dorsiflexion of the wrist and rotation of the forearm (Fig. 15.11). Clinically the condition may give rise to no symptoms, but there may be loss of strength in the wrist and sometimes pain on heavy use.

Radiographs show shortening and deformity of the radius with triangulation of its distal epiphysis and premature fusion of the ulna half of the distal radial growth plate (Fig. 15.12). The distal end of the ulna is subluxated dorsally and the proximal row of carpal bones have a triangular configuration with the lunate lying at the apex.

Bilateral Madelung deformity is a component of dyschondrosteosis but unilateral abnormality may follow trauma or occur as an isolated primary anomaly. Trauma may cause damage to the distal radial epiphysis before closure of the growth plate, resulting in premature fusion with consequent prominence of the head of the ulna. The triangulation of the radial epiphysis and carpus is not usually marked. The primary Madelung deformity is unilateral and non-genetic but otherwise similar to that seen in dyschondrosteosis.

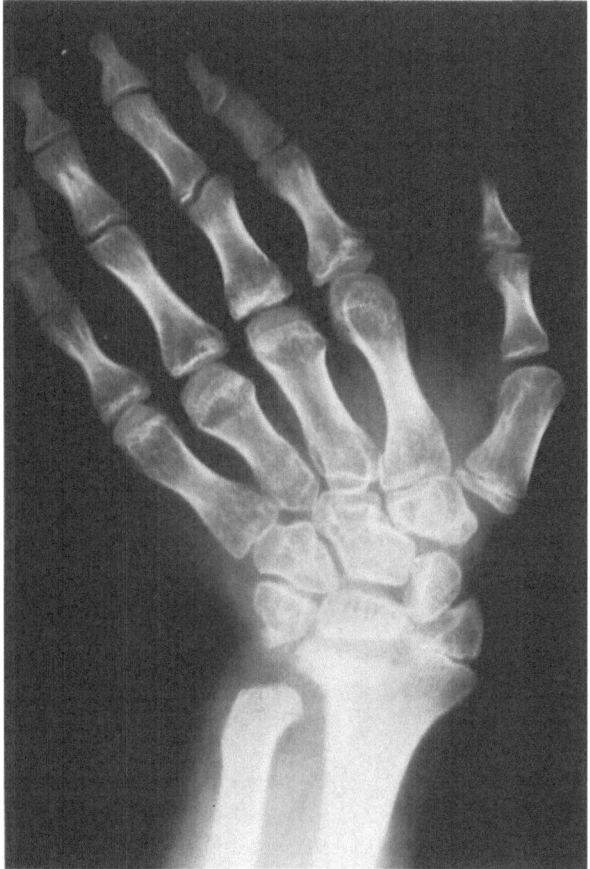

Fig. 15.11. Dyschondrosteosis. The Madelung deformity in a child.

Matev and Karangacheva (1975) described 12 patients with the primary deformity of whom four were males. Golding and Blackburne (1976) examined 26 patients with this abnormality in a survey in the West Indies, and since all were female the authors concluded that the primary deformity did not occur in the male, and that in previous reports of affected males the condition was due to dyschondrosteosis or trauma.

Management

The Madelung deformity does not generally interfere with function, but its appearance may cause concern. In these circumstances the head of the ulna can be excised and an osteotomy undertaken through the lower end of the radius to realign the carpus.

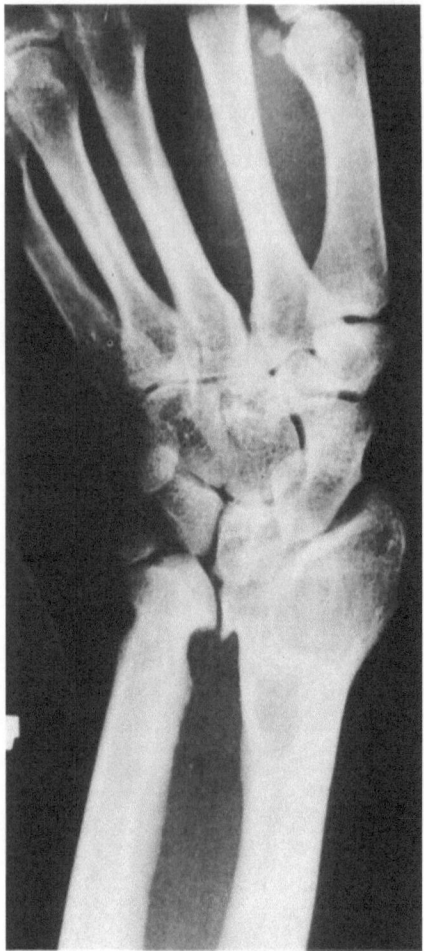

Fig. 15.12. Dyschondrosteosis. The Madelung deformity in an adult. Premature fusion of the ulnar half of the distal radial growth plate, subluxation of the lower end of the ulna and a triangular configuration of the proximal row of carpal bones.

15.11 Mesomelic Dysplasia

The mesomelic dysplasias are a group of inherited skeletal disorders and present clinically with dwarfism and limb shortening which is maximal in the forearms and the lower portion of the legs. These conditions are all rare and bear eponyms which include Langer, Nievergelt, Reinhardt-Pfeiffer and Werner. The different forms are distinguished by specific clinical and radiographic changes and by recognition of the characteristic pattern of inheritance. In acromesomelic dwarfism marked shortening of the digits is present in addition to the changes in the shanks and forearms (Fig. 15.13).

Apart from the problems caused by severe short stature, the general health is good in the mesomelic dysplasias. However, operation may be required for a Madelung deformity in the Langer form and for equinus feet and malaligned lower limbs in the Nievergelt type.

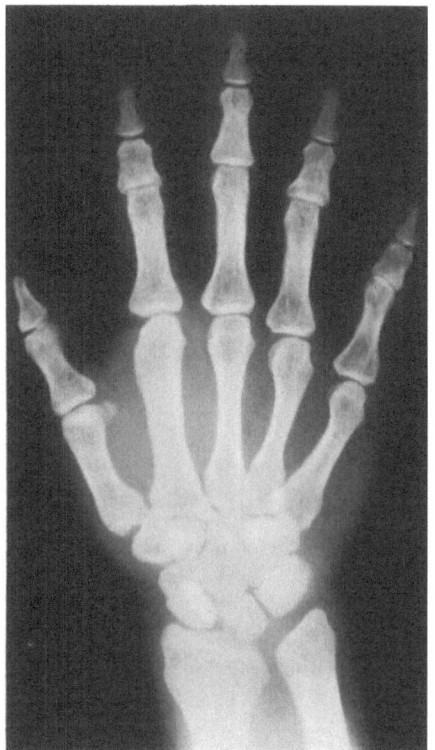

Fig. 15.13. Acromesomelic dwarfism. Radiograph of an adult hand.

References

Osteopoikilosis

Mindell ER, Cole S Northup, Douglas HO (1978) Osteosarcoma associated with osteopoikilosis. J Bone
  Joint Surg [Am] 60:406

Melorheostosis

Campbell CJ, Papademitrou T, Bonfiglio M (1968) Melorheostosis. A report of the clinical, roentgenog-
  raphic and pathological findings in fourteen cases. J Bone Joint Surg [Am] 50:1281
Young D, Drummond D, Herring J, Cruess RL (1979) Melorheostosis in children. J Bone Joint Surg [Br]
  61:415

Osteopathia Striata

Horan FT, Beighton PH (1978) Osteopathia striata with cranial sclerosis. An autosomal dominant entity.
  Clin Genet 13:201
Walker BA (1969) Osteopathia striata with cataracts and deafness. Birth Defects 5:295

Cleido-cranial Dysplasia

Fauré C, Maroteaux P (1973) Cleidocranial dysplasia. Progress in Pediatric Radiology [4]:211

Marfan Syndrome

Robins PR, Winter RB, Moe JH (1974) Scoliosis in patients with Marfan's syndrome. J Bone Joint Surg [Am] 56:1540

Homocystinuria

Thomas PS, Carson NAJ (1978) Homocystinuria. The evolution of skeletal changes in relation to treatment. Ann Radiol 21:95

Larsen Syndrome

Larsen LJ, Schottstaedt ER, Bost FD (1950) Multiple congenital dislocations associated with a characteristic facial abnormality. J Pediatr 37:574
Latta RJ, Graham CB, Aase JM, Scham SM, Smith DW (1971) Larsen's syndrome: a skeletal dysplasia with multiple joint dislocations and unusual facies. J Pediatr 78:291
Oki T, Terashima Y, Murachi S, Nogami H (1976) Clinical features and treatment of joint dislocations in Larsen's syndrome. Report of three cases in one family. Clin Orthop 119:206

Schwartz Syndrome

Horan F, Beighton P (1975) Orthopaedic aspects of the Schwartz syndrome. J Bone Joint Surg [Am] 57:542

Dyschondrosteosis

Golding JSR, Blackburne JS (1976) Madelung's disease of the wrist and dyschondrosteosis. J Bone Joint Surg [Br] 58B:350
Matev I, Karagancheva S (1975) The Madelung deformity. The Hand 7:152

Appendix

Textbooks, Monographs and Reviews Concerning Inherited Skeletal Dysplasias

Birth Defects Original Article Series, The National Foundation, March of Dimes. Editor D. Bergsma:
Limb Malformations, vol X, no. 5, 1974
Malformation Syndromes vol X, no. 7, 1974
Skeletal Dysplasias, vol X, no. 9, 1974
Skeletal Dysplasias, vol X, no. 12, 1974
Disorders of Connective Tissue, vol XI, no. 6, 1975
Morphogenesis and Malformation of the Limb, vol XIII, no. 1, 1977
The Genetics of Hand Malformations, vol XIV, no. 3, 1978

Bailey JA II (1973) Disproportionate short stature. Saunders, Philadelphia London Toronto
Beighton P (1978) Inherited disorders of the skeleton. Churchill Livingstone, Edinburgh London New York
Beighton P, Cremin BJ (1980) Sclerosing bone dysplasias. Springer, Berlin Heidelberg New York
Bergsma D (ed) (1979) Birth defects compendium 2nd edn. Alan R. Liss, New York (The National Foundation-March of Dimes)
Carter CO, Fairbank TJ (1974) The genetics of locomotor disorders. Oxford University Press, London New York Toronto
Cremin BJ, Beighton P (1978) Bone dysplasias of infancy. Springer, Berlin Heidelberg New York
Gorlin RJ, Pindborg JP, Cohen MM Jr (1976) Syndromes of the head and neck, 2nd edn. McGraw-Hill, London New York Toronto
Kaufman HJ (ed) (1973) Intrinsic diseases of bones. Karger, Basel München Paris New York Sydney (Progress in pediatric radiology, vol 4)
Maroteaux P (1979) Bone diseases of children. Lippincott, Philadelphia, Toronto
McKusick VA (1972) Heritable disorders of connective tissue, 4th edn. Mosby, St Louis
McKusick VA (1978) Mendelian inheritance in man, 5th edn. Johns Hopkins Press, Baltimore London
Smith DW (1976) Recognizable patterns of human malformations, 2nd edn. Saunders, Philadelphia London Toronto
Spranger JW, Langer LO, Wiedemann H-R (1974) Bone dysplasias. Fischer, Stuttgart
Warkany J (1971) Congenital malformations. Year Book Medical Publishers, Chicago
Wynne-Davies R, Fairbank TJ (1976) Fairbank's Atlas of general affections of the skeleton, 2nd edn. Churchill Livingstone, Edinburgh London New York

Subject Index

B. J. Cremin, P. Beighton

Bone Dysplasias of Infancy

A Radiological Atlas

Foreword from R. O. Murray
1978. 55 figures in 124 separate illustrations,
4 tables. XIII, 109 pages
ISBN 3-540-08816-4

Contents: Clinical and Genetic Evaluation of the
Neonate with Skeletal Dysplasia. – Radiographic
Techniques. – Achondrogenesis. – Thanatophoric
Dysplasia. – Asphyxiating Thoracic Dysplasia. –
Chondroectodermal Dysplasia. – Lethal Short Rib-
Polydactyly Syndromes. – Chondrodysplasia
Punctata. – Campomelic Dysplasia. – Achondro-
plasia. – Diastrophic Dysplasia. – Metatropic Dys-
plasia. – Spondyloepiphyseal Dysplasia Con-
genita. – Mesomelic Dysplasia. – Larsen Syn-
drome. – Cleido-Cranial Dysplasia. – Osteogenesis
Imperfecta Congenita. – Hypophosphatasia. –
Osteopetrosis and Other Sclerosing Bone Dys-
plasias.

from the reviews:
"The recent explosion of publications on general
skeletal dysplasias is continued in this admirable
and profusely illustrated little book emanating from
the Departments of Radiology and of Human
Genetics in the University of Cape Town. Its origins
set the tone, the main emphasis falling on the radiological appearances, these being the most important
diagnostic feature in infancy, and on the prognosis,
especially the genetic prognosis, so that whenever
possible the parents may receive suitable counselling. The book is especially directed towards those
in training in the radiology of the newborn, but is
of equal importance to obstetricians and paedia-
tricians, and also to orthopaedic surgeons whose
opinion may be sought... a most successful venture
and a useful reference book on a subject un-
commonly seen outside specialist units; we look
forward to further contributions from this very progressive school."
The Journal of Bone and Joint Surgery

"The authors point out the field has not as yet been
completely explored. But what they do present not
only indicates the value of many new diagnostic
techniques in the early recognition of these disorders, but offers an accurate prognosis for many of
these affected children."
Orthopaedic Review

P. Beighton, B. J. Cremin

Sclerosing Bone Dysplasias

Foreword by H. G. Jacobson
1980. 62 figures in 218 separate illustrations.
IX, 191 pages
ISBN 3-540-09471-7

Contents: Introduction. – History and Nomencla-
ture. – Clinical and Genetic Aspects. – Radiologic
Considerations. – Osteopetrosis. – Pycnodysosto-
sis. – Metaphyseal Dysplasia (Pyle Disease) –
Craniometaphyseal Dysplasia. – Craniodiaphyseal
Dysplasia. – Frontometaphyseal Dysplasia. –
Osteodysplasty (Melnick-Needles Syndrome). –
Dysosteosclerosis. – Endosteal Hyperostosis. –
Sclerosteosis. – Diaphyseal Dysplasia (Camurati-
Engelmann Disease). – Osteopathia Striata. –
Osteopoikilosis. – Melorheostosis. – Osteoectasia
with Hyperphosphatasia. – Infantile Cortical
Hyperostosis (Caffey Disease). – Oculodento-
Osseous Dysplasia. – Miscellaneous Sclerosing
Dysplasias. – Differential Diagnosis: Other
Sclerosing Disorders. – Subject Index.

from the reviews:
"Professors Beighton and Cremin have done it
again! The University of Cape Town team of medical
geneticist and radiologist have produced another
excellent book, which is a worthy successor to their
Bone Dysplasias of Infancy published in 1978 and
widely acclaimed. No fewer than 17 sclerosing bone
dysplasias are treated in separate chapters under the
headings historical and nosological considerations,
clinical features, radiographic manifestations, and
comment. At the end of each chapter there is a list
of useful references as well as a number of illustrations of high-quality radiographs and, where appropriate, clinical photographs. Some chapters contain
tables which will prove extremely useful in dis-
tinguishing one disease from another, or even the
autosomal dominant form of a condition from the
recessive type."
South African Medical Journal

"Beighton and Cremin have combined their skills
in genetics and radiology to write a fascinating book
on sclerosing bone dysplasias. The area is small, and
so is the book (191 pages). However, the coverage
appears to be complete and the discussions are
concise and easy to read. The illustrations are of
excellent technical quality and include both radiographs and pertinent clinical photographs. The
references are more than adequate."
The Journal of Bone and Joint Surgery

"...for the person who is interested in the less
common orthopedic disorders, and particularly for
the pediatric orthopedist, this volume represents a
quantum leap in clarity and well-organized
content."
Orthopedics

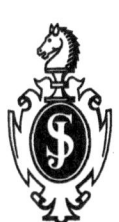

Springer-Verlag Berlin Heidelberg New York

F. Schajowicz

Tumors and Tumorlike Lesions of Bone and Joints

1981. 948 figures, 2 color inserts.
XIV, 581 pages
ISBN 3-540-90492-1
Distribution rights for Japan:
Nankodo Co., Tokyo

W. Blauth, F. Schneider-Sickert

Congenital Deformities of the Hand

An Atlas of Their Surgical Treatment

Translated from the German by U. H. Weil
1981. 426 figures (most in color).
XV, 387 pages
ISBN 3-540-10084-9

H. A. Keim

The Adolescent Spine

With contributions by J. R. Denton,
H. M. Dick, J. G. McMurtry, III, D. P. Roye, Jr.
2nd edition. 1982. 366 figures. XV, 254 pages
ISBN 3-540-90612-6

E. Somerville

Displacement of the Hip in Childhood

Aetiology, Management and Sequelae

1982. 262 figures. XIII, 200 pages
ISBN 3-540-10936-6

A. Wackenheim, E. Babin

The Narrow Lumbar Canal

Radiologic Signs and Surgery

With a Foreword by L. Jeanmart
1980. 139 figures in 292 separate illustrations,
7 tables. XIII, 170 pages
ISBN 3-540-09443-1

P. Doury, Y. Dirheimer, S. Pattin

Algodystrophy

Diagnosis and Therapy of a Frequent Disease
of the Locomotor Apparatus

With a Foreword by J. Villiaumey
Translated from the French by
M.-T. Wackenheim
1981. 46 figures. XVI, 165 pages
ISBN 3-540-10624-3

Segmental Idiopathic Necrosis of the Femoral Head

Editor: U. H. Weil
With contributions numerous experts

1981. 68 figures, 30 tables. VII, 121 pages
(Progress in Orthopedic Surgery, Volume 5)
ISBN 3-540-10718-5

Springer-Verlag
Berlin
Heidelberg
New York

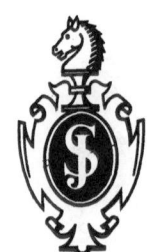